TOXIC
BI

C000042642

BILL KELLNER-READ

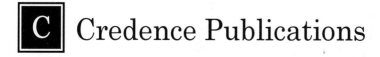 Credence Publications

First published in 2002
by Credence Publications

ISBN 1-904015-00-X

Printed and bound in the UK by
Credence Publications
PO Box 3
TONBRIDGE
Kent TN12 9ZY
England
www.credence.org

Cover design by S Ransom

1st ed. GN

Table of Contents

"It is with great pleasure that I write this brief testimonial for my good friend and colleague Bill Kellner-Read. My first encounter with Bill was in the treatment of a mutual patient who was suffering from acute head pain. Together, using a combination of dental plane corrections, cranial, cervical and spinal adjustments, we were able to solve this lady's problems. This was one of those typical cases where the lady had been everywhere, seen all the specialists, spent thousands of dollars and got nowhere. It was after this success that we started a long and productive professional relationship.

Bill is a very creative, lateral-thinking man who does not accept the status quo. This attitude has gained him much respect both from his professional colleagues and the thousands of people he has helped over the years.

A thinker, a developer and a gifted man who is always looking for ways to better help humanity, I know that you, the reader, will gain much valuable information from Bill's book. And if you apply the information, then it will help you to a healthier, happier lifestyle." **Michael Troy D.C. (Doctor of Chiropractic), Queensland, Australia**

"I have known Bill Kellner-Read for nearly fifteen years and have greatly admired him for the way that he has relentlessly pursued knowledge. Bill has achieved a real understanding of the rights and many wrongs in dentistry. He has travelled the world in the search for answers to important questions and, as a result of being a great student, has become a great teacher. He has shared his knowledge with colleagues and many others in various areas of health care. Bill was one of the first to realise that by combining the modalities of dentistry with chiropractic, physiotherapy, osteopathy and various other treatment modalities, he could achieve a much higher standard of care for his patients." **Dr Simon Coggin B.D.S.(Dental Surgeon), Australia.**

"Bill's image of himself as a dentist encompasses a far greater range of ideas than I, and I am sure most of my colleagues have *envisaged. He has involved me in his interest in the control of chronic pain, which is a major part of his practice. I feel Bill's experience and knowledge of the diagnosis and treatment of temporo-mandibular joint dysfunction and associated chronic pain problems make him an invaluable asset in the community."* **Dr John Casey B.D.S.(NZ), Dental Surgeon, New Zealand.**

"I have been practising dentistry for 16 years. I started working with Bill Kellner-Read about 18 months ago. I was enthralled by his level of knowledge, enthusiasm and passion for his chosen path in dentistry.

At that time I had been suffering with severe headaches. I discussed these with Bill and I became aware that he might be able to help with this problem. He made me a splint and the headaches disappeared, "never to raise their ugly heads again."

Since that time I have been free from headaches, thanks to Bill. In my sixteen years in practice, I have never come across any dentist who has the ability and compassion shown by Bill. I wish there were more people of his calibre.

His work and ideas have shown me that there is much more to offer than we were taught at dental school. I can now understand that problems I looked at from a purely dental aspect are more than likely multi-factorial.

There is so much that we as yet still don't know and it is with this in mind that I am so pleased that Bill has written this book. While it is essentially for the lay-person, I believe that it will open the eyes of many in my profession of dentistry. I do hope so!" **Dr Nikki McBlain. B.D.S. (Edinburgh)**

Introduction

I'm the guy you wait to see as you flip through those *National Geographic* and *Saga* magazines in the dentist's waiting room, the cold knot of dread tightening in your stomach as you tune in to assorted drills whining away down the gleaming, white corridor. I see you stiffen in 'as relaxed and casual a way as possible' as you enter my den. I am an expert at body language. I note your trepidation as you glance nervously at my instruments of torture – instruments that trigger the universally-shared response of *"Lord, get me out of here!"* Instruments that, upon first glance even, have the power to pepper your memory cells with ghastly and everlasting imagery.

Metallic, glinting instruments that poke, prod, scrape and make those ear-piercing, 'fingernails-down-the-blackboard' sounds, sending shivers down your spine. Chemical compounds that are supposed to assist in ridding your teeth of cavities, prolonging the life of that single molar at the back, better known as Juanita (One-Eater), and granting a reprieve from the executioner's forceps. Chemicals that reduce inflammation, desensitise the teeth and remedy the many other unfortunate afflictions of the mouth. All these tools and more do I have at my disposal.

We dentists are also in the loop with every new technical innovation that comes onto the market in the sphere of dental health and hygiene. And we get to try most of this new stuff out on you too. But the old kit is the best. We have the overhead lights, we have the X-ray machine, and of course, the drill!

So from 8:30 in the morning until the wife's patience gives out and our dinner ends up inside the family pet, it's Lights! Camera! Action! What's it like being a dentist? Long hours. Painstaking work. A bit like mending the roads, only no traffic lights.

My consuming interest for many years has been in health. Why is it that some people just don't get sick? The more stalwart among us maybe suffer the occasional cold, even the beginnings of flu, but these afflictions seem miraculously to fade before the illness has a chance to take hold. But for others - total wipe-out for a few days, sometimes a few weeks. Many of us suffer throughout our lives, moving seamlessly from one ailment to another. Those incessant trips to the doctor. More prescriptions, more drugs, more time off work.

LIVE FOREVER

And then, while some people never suffer bad teeth, gum disease or need orthodontics, others dwell permanently on the waiting lists of their local dental office. How is it that backaches, headaches and neckaches ruin people's lives, and yet others seem to be able to eat, drink and smoke too much and almost live forever?

Today dentistry is embroiled in controversy just like all other branches of medicine, and indeed has been ever since the first dentist attached a piece of string to a tooth and looped the other end to the tail of a fast and angry horse. Should we take vitamins and minerals to improve dental health, or are we just excreting expensive urine? Does mercury cause neurological diseases or is it really a non-toxic metal used in dental fillings? Does sodium fluoride in your toothpaste help in the battle against tooth decay, or is it a toxin that increases the risk of hip fracture and cancer? And what of sugar? Is tooth decay sugar's only indictment, or is it, as has been reported, one of the most damaging substances we can put into our body?

After some years in general dental practice, I began noticing an uncomfortable shifting in my views, based on an increasing amount of contrary scientific evidence which appeared to demonstrate that a significant portion of dental practice was harming the patient.

ENTRENCHED SCIENTIFIC ERROR

I discovered that many treatments available from a standard dental clinic today are based on entrenched scientific error as well as a fundamental, erroneous assumption of what caused the dental problem to begin with. I also uncovered surprising evidence that some of the most basic tenets underpinning dentistry are flawed - and even worse, downright dangerous. Could it be possible that mercury amalgams, root canals, fluoride pastes, and others were benefiting the chemical industry more than the patient? And what of the burgeoning profits made from dentistry? Was there a connection between the levels of rotten teeth, gingivitis and bad breath consistently showing up in the neighbourhood, and the amount of paper whirring through the dental office credit card machine? Was this a simple but unsettling case of sickness meaning big business?

Realistically, overall dental health in many societies today is not better than it was two decades ago. In fact, it's worse. And this is not necessarily because of the dentist's inability to fix the problems; we have at our disposal fantastic state of the art equipment and procedures to solve even the most complex of cases. The bottom-line is two-fold: the public hasn't learned to give up abusing their bodies with food, and the dentist hasn't learned to give up inflicting abuse on his patients caused by some of his treatments. There simply are no realistic, consistent efforts being made by dental medicine to prevent dental problems from occurring in our society in the first place.

There's the passing lip-service paid to *'Sugar is Very Naughty, Young Malcolm'* and the myriad toothpaste ads that claim *'8 out of 10 Dentists Recommend It'*. This of course got me wondering what happened to the other two who didn't *'recommend it'*. What were their reasons? As we shall discover, the toothpaste industry represents very big business. Is it possible that those two dissenters were not prepared to be intellectually 'bought out'? Were they perhaps showing certain resistance to some of the industry's whiter-than-white toothpaste folklore?

PROFESSIONAL PRIDE
Dentistry is a pride thing too. I know my work is examined by other professionals and I in turn examine their handiwork when it passes my way. What are my views on the art of my dental colleagues? As in any profession, you have the sculptors and then you have the quarry-blasters and road-menders. Not that there is anything wrong with these last two noble professions when applied to mining and highways. It's only wrong when you find evidence of their art in the mouth of the patient. It's as simple as this: what you don't know about your teeth could possibly lead to your premature demise. The danger which threatens every member of society today

is not readily traced back to the dentist's chair, and yet could it be possible that millions of people around the world have already been killed or maimed by the inadvertent or deliberate application of certain dental techniques that have come to be regarded in our cultures today as beyond reproach.

TOOTHACHE LORD

Toothache is as old as time itself. We have looked for cures for this age-old problem; pills, potions, tinctures - many of which would cause more harm than good. Perhaps no stranger case of toothache exists than that of the Toothache Lord of St. Stephan's Cathedral in Vienna. This splendid cathedral rises up like a coral reef from the sea of buildings in the inner city of Vienna. Since the days of its construction, it has served as a symbol of the history and destiny of Austria itself. On the west wall of the tower chamber of the North Tower stands the original bust of a Gothic Man of Sorrows named *"Toothache Lord."* The name stems from the following legend:

Drunken men on their way home from a night of carousing walked through St. Stephan's churchyard and made fun of the facial expression of the Man of Sorrows, hooting *"The Lord has a toothache."* They tied a cloth around the head and mocked him. During the night they were struck with severe toothache and only after they had made a pilgrimage to the Toothache Lord to beg forgiveness did their pains subside.

Of course dentists aren't so forgiving. Imagine, there you are, in a dental surgery in downtown Vienna looking for forgiveness for your weekend of revelry on Goesser beer, coffee and cakes. You sit in the confessional, which doubles as a dental chair, and open your mouth wide to receive forgiveness.

MILKING THE TOOTH

The blunt end of the mirror is inserted into the oral cavity to tap the offending tooth. The pain reaches a crescendo and they peel you from the ceiling. Back in the chair, they tap the offending tooth once more to make sure they have found the right one. This is called tender-to-percussion and denotes an abscess at the tip of the root - tender, of course, being a dental understatement for excruciating agony. The offending tooth is drilled to gain relief, pus and dead nerve tissue are removed, the root canal is attended to and a filling in the tooth completes the procedure.

Of course, this is not the end. The tooth becomes brittle and before it breaks, it needs a crown. This is as far as it goes, until the pain recurs and the treatment procedure is repeated *ad infinitum*, or until the tooth is finally extracted – whatever the patient's wishes.

DOC HOLLIDAY

You could have been treated by the infamous 'Doc Holliday'. John Henry Holliday attended the Pennsylvania College of Dental Surgery, Philadelphia in 1869.[1] At the age of 20, he was awarded the Doctor of Dental Surgery degree and promptly set off for Dallas. He was welcomed for his skill as he replaced the local blacksmith who had two choices of treatment: extraction or extraction.

Indeed Doc was a good dentist who shared top prize in several categories of dental craftsmanship at the annual North Texas Fair. Unfortunately he had been diagnosed with tuberculosis and it was his coughing that made his patients uncomfortable rather than his skill. And it is not so different nowadays. There is nothing worse then treating a patient when you've got a cold. There they are, their mouth nine inches away from your nose, when it starts to run. They attempt in vain to turn the head or close the mouth, only to be told to stay still and keep the mouth open, the dentist believing that they are wriggling in pain, while in fact they are trying to avoid the drop of nasal fluid about to descend into the open mouth. But I digress.

SHOOT OUT!

Disgruntled by his continual health problems, Doc Holliday turned to liquor and gambling. This led to his first salon shoot-out in 1875. This made him a dangerous dentist. If you didn't like his treatment, you got shot. It is fair to say, in any case, that John

---

[1] Heynick, Frank, "How to Drill a Man in More Ways Than One", *Dentistry*, 17th May 2001, www.doc-holliday.net

Henry Holliday was a dentist who knew how to drill a man in more ways than one.

AIR FORCE DENTIST

I went for an interview to become a dentist in the Air Force. I enquired about periodontal abscesses, the cleaning of the teeth and resolution of the problem. *"Problem? What problem?"* said the Captain. *"There is no problem. We just take out the tooth and keep them flying. We've spent a great deal on their training. Can't let a spot of toothache get in the way!"*

Hopefully, things might have changed a bit by now!

Dentistry has also been practiced in its basic form on and off the rugby fields of England. I remember removing two teeth from the back of my brother's head and having to take his poor opponent down to the surgery to have his fractured front teeth root-filled. On another occasion, Len, a team-mate of mine, came up to me in the bar after a game, complaining of toothache. We'd had a couple of beers and neither of us wanted to leave, so we decided that when we were ready we would try to remove his tooth there and then in the club-house. It didn't seem to matter how many beers he had consumed, the pain persisted.

Now, don't get me wrong. I liked Len. But it's irritating when toothache gets in the way of a good beer and the sing-song that graces most rugby clubs on a Saturday night. I'd had enough, so I recruited a couple of guys to hold him down while I removed the culprit with my fingers (not to be attempted at home without a safety net!). The big boys turned away in disgust, their usual ruddy complexion for once replaced by a deathly pallor. Len, with relief in his eyes and a smile on his face, bought me another beer for my trouble.

CROWNING BEAUTY?

One of my earliest 'dental' memories is of a school dance. I was with a beautiful girl who had acrylic crowns. She looked fantastic until the UV lights switched on. She turned and smiled at me. Her front teeth were missing. The acrylic crowns did not reflect the light and so she had a black hole where her front teeth used to be. I can't remember what I said but she's only just begun talking to me again after thirty years.

TEETHING TROUBLES

Over the years, children haven't fared much better. Teething has been held responsible for a wide variety of childhood illnesses.[2] There are references to teething difficulties in Homeric hymns from around 1200 BC and in the prayers of early Indian literature around 100 BC. This from Hippocrates, taken from his short treatise entitled *On Dentition*:

"Teething children suffer from itching of the gums, fevers, convulsions and diarrhoea, especially when they cut their eye teeth and when they are very corpulent and costive." [3]

Here is a recorded cure from the fourth century AD:

"If they are in pain, smear the gums with dog's milk or hare's brain; this works also if eaten. But if a tooth is coming through with difficulty, smear Cyperas with butter and oil-of-lilies over the part where it is erupting." [4]

Ambroise Pare (1517–1592), the French army surgeon, began to advocate a new solution to the age-old problem of breeding teeth: cutting the gums with a lancet. In 1575, he described how he developed the method, from the examination of a dead child.

"When we diligently sought for the cause of his death, we could impute it to nothing else than the contumacious hardness of the gums... when we cut the gums with a knife we found all the teeth appearing... if it had been done when he lived, doubtless he would have been preserved." [5]

Dr. Ashley concludes his paper by saying:

---

[2] Ashley, M P, "It's Only Teething. A Report on the Myths and Modern Approaches to Teething", *British Dental Journal*, Vol. 191, No.1, July 2001
[3] Hippocrates, *On Dentition: 25th Aphorism*, 3rd book, 4th Century BC
[4] Ashley, M P, "It's Only Teething...", ibid.
[5] Ashley, M P, ibid.

"The beliefs and superstitions associated with teething throughout history appear amusing and it may cause concern that the profession was so willing to go along with practices so incorrect. Yet it is sobering to appreciate that our historic colleagues were acting on their existing knowledge and their professional and personal standing relied heavily on their reputation amongst their peers and patients. Maybe things have not changed so much after all. Will our colleagues of the future be smirking at our misguided ways?"[6]

MISGUIDED

Amusing though these anecdotes may be, the question is, should our present-day willingness to go along with incorrect practices be cause for concern? Over 150 years ago, mercury fillings gained acceptance amongst the dental profession. There we were, putting in the mercury because it was easy to use, effective and cheap. As time went by, this unbelievable practice became accepted. Today we are still using this neurotoxin as a filling material. Misguided? Perhaps tomorrow our peers may smirk at us for having used mercury, raising their eyes to heaven in absolute disbelief that we could have used such a product. Time will tell.

DARK AGES

In actual fact, dentistry has a great deal to offer, as anyone who has suffered toothache will admit. I wouldn't want to go back to the dark ages of tooth-pulling or having a hole punched into my skull to relieve the agonising pain of a headache. Sound dental intervention has given relief from pain for millions of people over the years. It is not the dentistry that is questioned so much as the effect on the human frame as a result of the materials used.

NO FEAR!

The dental surgery is no longer a place to be feared. The sophistication and innovation of dentists around the world have made this profession far less foreboding than it was even twenty years ago. Even for the most fearful, there are techniques that can reduce the trauma of the visit to an absolute minimum. The drills

---

[6] Ashley, M P, ibid.

are of the finest, with speeds that make tooth cutting a swift and relatively painless experience. As a profession, we are ever improving in technique and patient-focussed consideration.

This book highlights many of those changes that have been made or need to be implemented. It looks at the downside but also gives hope to millions of sufferers who still go from specialist to specialist looking for answers that perhaps can only be found sitting in the dentist's chair.

Thank you for choosing to read **Toxic Bite**.

Stressors and How We Get Sick

The American Cancer Society is quoted as saying that currently around 590,000 Americans die from cancer annually and this figure is expected to rise dramatically every year.[7] What this has to do with the root fillings you receive, the dentures you wear or the gum disease which makes your teeth so mobile or your breath at best 'not sweet' is not immediately apparent. But cancer and dental health are indeed directly and intricately linked.

Research shows that advanced gum disease may lead to heart disease, respiratory disorders and pre-term, low-weight babies.[8] Root fillings may cause systemic disease in different organs of the body. The fluoride in your toothpaste can cause dental fluorosis or an increase in hip fracture, while mercury fillings may be responsible for multiple sclerosis and other neurological disorders. We will be examining all of these factors in more detail in the following pages.

STRESS!

Hans Selye, the Austrian endocrinologist and researcher, is quoted as saying that accumulated bad news rots the whole apple. Actually he didn't. He said:

"Stress is the non-specific reaction of the body to any demand placed upon it."[9]

Stress is also cumulative. The more garbage you put into or onto the body, the more chance your body will creak under the strain and the more you will move from ease to dis-ease. With cancer currently afflicting around one in three in the UK and heart disease still the leading killer, it might make sense to start looking at the garbage.

---

[7] Day, Phillip, *Cancer: Why We're Still Dying to Know the Truth*, Credence, 2001

[8] Academy of Periodontology, www.perio.org/consumer/mbc.top2.htm

[9] Selye, Hans, *Stress Without Distress*, Signet, New American Library, 1975

WHAT IS CANCER?

American biochemist Ernst T Krebs Jr. produced his landmark thesis fifty years ago, which demonstrated that cancer is a healing process that simply hasn't terminated upon completion of its task.[10] When we are damaged by environmental contaminants (carcinogens), our bodies initiate a healing process to fix the damage. In the event of our having depressed immune systems and nutrition deficiencies, these healing processes may not terminate, giving rise to an uncontrolled proliferation of stem-cell trophoblast (healing material) within our bodies that is later identified as a cancer.

Krebs went on to pioneer a fascinating, non-patentable treatment for cancer, which has received the approbation and endorsement of some of the most experienced names in science. The treatment is designed to terminate the spread of this trophoblastic expansion and consists entirely of food materials and nutritive elements.

Not surprisingly, Krebs' Metabolic Therapy incurred the wrath of the conventional medical establishment which viewed unpatentable raw materials, available in any supermarket, as a threat to the $200 billion a year cancer industry.[11]

ADVICE ON DIET

Cancer prevention operates on two principles: Pack the body with nutrition, together with bolstering the immune system and disease-fighting capabilities of the human organism with an active, healthy lifestyle. And secondly, avoid taking in, and being surrounded with toxins that can cause damage to the body. Every good sports club provides programs to reduce excess weight and get

---

[10] Krebs, Ernst T, *B17 Metabolic Therapy, a technical manual*, Credence, 2002

[11] For a full report on Krebs' work with cancer and an in-depth investigation into the merits of Metabolic Therapy, please see Day, Phillip, *Cancer: Why We're Still Dying to Know the Truth*, Credence Publications, 2001; *B17 Metabolic Therapy – a technical manual*, Credence Publications, 2002. Clinical applications of this amazing and simple protocol are also reported in Griffin, G Edward, *World Without Cancer*, and Binzel, Philip, *Alive & Well*, American Media, 2000 (also available through Credence Publications). Dr Binzel has used Metabolic Therapy for cancer treatment for over thirty years with remarkable results.

the blood coursing through those cobwebby veins. Adhering to a good exercise regime results in lower blood pressure and heart rate, increased oxygen in the body, a movable lymph system and stronger immunity to disease. The end result of course, is better health, less disease, more energy and a healthier, happier existence. So, are we prepared to do what it takes?

"He who does not use his endeavours to heal himself is brother to him who commits suicide." Proverbs 18:9 (Amplified Bible)

We are singularly and wonderfully made, each one of us uniquely different, yet, at a cellular level, the same, with similar cellular requirements. I need the same vitamins, minerals and trace elements as you to make a cell. If I don't have enough, I can't make good cells. If I don't have good cells, then I don't have a healthy body. If environmental toxins are continually damaging my cells or my nutrition is poor and I have a poor immune response, then potentially I could be in big trouble with cancer and other degenerative diseases.

If I continue to put carcinogens onto or into my body, use toxins in my toothpaste and drink sugar water masquerading as lemonade, then at some time in the future, I will receive the sure reward for my consistent and health-damaging efforts. I'm going to get a disease.

STRESS AND THE MEDICAL MODEL

When I first looked at stress, I thought that it was nervous tension. And it would appear that my medical colleagues concurred. I would have patients in my surgery telling me that they suffered stress - a nervous tension that was all in the mind. They were given Valium or Prozac by their physicians and told to go home, relax and learn to live with it. They were suffering head, neck and back pain, earache, ringing in the ears, insomnia, irritable bowel, painful periods, emotional irritability, thyroid problems, elevated blood pressure, high cholesterol and more – the list is endless. All would appear to be due to this nervous tension.

The stressors that afflict us can be physical, chemical, structural, emotional and environmental. The brain responds by producing elevated levels of neurotransmitter hormones, such as adrenaline, to prepare us physically and mentally to meet the challenge. Stress becomes cumulative if not discharged. So does the constant hormone activity caused by the stress, which in turn, precipitates the releasing of sugars, insulin, vitamin and mineral depletion and dehydration, which leads to physical and mental degeneration and disease. Selye called this the General Adaptation Syndrome. This GAS comprises three distinct phases.

THE ALARM REACTION

The first stage is fight or flight.[12] Either you stand and fight or you run away. This is when you feel the thumping heart, your hands go cold and clammy, and you get nervous (the well-known effects of the neurotransmitter adrenaline). This is the reaction before a big race, an exam or the first date. It is quite normal and after the stimulus has gone, everything should return to normal. Unfortunately things in life are not always this simple. Unwanted stresses are cumulative, rather like filling a bucket with water. Imagine you are this bucket and life stresses are flowing into your bucket. Instead of emptying the bucket, you allow it to fill - one stress upon another. As each stress is added, you lose the ability to return to normal. Instead you build up a resistance to these stresses.

RESISTANCE

In the second stage, our bodies instinctively cope with stresses as they accumulate. This is how most of us live our adult lives. Stresses build up through childhood and our teens. As they arrive, we deal with some and eliminate them, while others are stored. When we are young, fit and healthy, we can cope. Of course, this is not true for everybody. Some people seem to be born with their bucket three-quarters full.

While we live with a higher level of accumulated stress, we tell ourselves that this is part of life's rich tapestry and so we learn to live with it. We adapt and as each additional stressor is introduced, we file it away, take it on board, keep it or eliminate it. Our bodies

---

[12] Read, Bill, *A Bucketful of Stress*, 1993. Now available through the author c/o Credence Publications, PO Box 3, Tonbridge, Kent, TN12 9ZY, UK

are still producing hormones, such as insulin and adrenaline, to maintain the fight or flight impulse as each stressor arrives. Naturally, if we continue to add stresses, all the while eliminating less and less of them and their attendant hormonal effects on us, than we will go into overflow. The result is exhaustion, diseases such as heart disease and type 2 diabetes and even total body shutdown.[13]

EXHAUSTION

Stage three is when the body can no longer cope. It begins shutting itself down as an emergency precautionary measure to stop additional stressors entering and doing serious damage. The experience of a breakdown is well known to many: *"I don't know what happened, I was cruising through life and now, all of a sudden, I can't cope. I'm angry, emotional, can't make decisions, can't think, can't concentrate, can't face it any more. I'm more tired when I wake up in the morning than when I go to bed. I'm sick and tired of feeling sick and tired. My body hurts and I feel absolutely lousy."*

Overload, heart attack, stroke, ulcer, cancer, thyroid problems, diabetes, chronic pain, multiple allergies and hormonal disturbances will be the sure result if the patient does not re-prioritise his life and quick! Rest, recuperation, change in diet, hydration and supplementation are all part of the recovery process. But the patient has to *want* to do it. Mortuaries are full of proud workaholics.

MINERAL DEFICIENCY

Whilst stress can arise due to a life circumstance, this is not always the case. Stress can arrive due to a lack of essential minerals, vitamins and trace elements. All the bad guys are coming to get you but you don't have any good guys fighting for you. You haven't the building blocks of good nutrition to enable your body to build good cells and a healthy, robust immune system capable of dealing with the onslaught. It is at this point that we turn ·instinctively to the

---

[13] Day, Phillip, *Health Wars*, Credence, 2001. *Health Wars* gives us the bigger picture on the effects of compound stress and how we can cope and thrive under these circumstances.

conventional pharmacy to bail us out. Drugs are copiously prescribed to treat the symptoms, the overload and any other manifestations – but this is all that the drugs do - they treat the symptoms. They do not cure the underlying cause of the problem. In his book *The Dental Physician*, Aelred Fonder DDS, states:

"A drug may create a mistaken sense of well-being, but it neither affects nor corrects the underlying disease process which will continue slowly to fester and develop, if causation is not eliminated." [14]

BENEFICIAL INCOME OVER BENEFICIAL OUTCOME?

We already know the cause of many degenerative diseases. So why does the medical profession ignore these facts? Does the dispensing of drugs ensure a more stable income than teaching proper nutrition? Dental research specialist Dr Weston Price's research evidence clearly indicated the absence of something rather than the presence of something. The absence in question is the lack of good nutrition.

EMPTY FOODS

Then there's the *'Why fruit and veg were better for us 50 years ago'* headline in the Daily Mail, 5th March 2001. According to research reported in this paper, modern farming methods mean that the amount of essential minerals in the food we eat has been reduced alarmingly. There is up to 75% less calcium and 93% less copper in fruit and vegetables, the study reports. Runner beans, which used to contain a significant amount of sodium - vital for the working of nerves and muscles and the alkalising of the body, now have almost no traces of the mineral at all. The levels of other important nutrients such as iron, potassium and magnesium have also plummeted. Nutritionist David Thomas, who heads up the organisation Trace Minerals (UK), is one of many who has tabulated the results of government findings over the years regarding the mineral depletion of the soils. It makes for sobering reading.

---

[14] Fonder, Aelred, *The Dental Physician*, Medical-Dental Arts, 303 West 2nd Street, Rock Falls, 61071, USA, 1985

NO MINERALS

We need minerals and trace elements for the body to function. While farming has doubtless improved yield, it has done so at the expense of natural remineralisation of the soil. If the minerals are not in the soil, then they are not in the vegetation. These minerals are not synthesised by the plants but taken up by them from the soils. This accounts for our empty vegetables. It looks like a carrot, it smells like a carrot, it tastes like a carrot but it is empty of the magnesium necessary for protection against heart attacks, asthma and kidney stones.[15]

HEART DISEASE

The Lancet reports that the Caerphilly heart disease study of men aged between 45-59 provided evidence that low dietary magnesium is predictive of ischaemic heart disease.[16] Linus Pauling and Matthias Rath are world-famous for their work on heart disease, showing that a fulminating deficiency of Vitamin C in industrialised societies, coupled with a further reduction of existing Vitamin C levels due to smoking, stress and drugs, was causing the collagen fibres in our arteries to tear.

Pauling and Rath show how the body attempts to heal damaged arteries using lipoprotein (a). This accumulates like so many temporary band-aids, causing plaque build-up, atherosclerosis and further heart complaints.[17]

CHOCOLATE.... AND ME A DENTIST!

Magnesium-rich foods include nuts, shellfish, legumes, grain, dried fruits, dark leafy green vegetables and, I hate to say it as a

---

[15] See section entitled "Why Are the Nations Dying?"

[16] The Caerphilly Heart Disease Study, *The Lancet*, Vol. 340, 22nd August 1992

[17] Rath, Matthias, *Why Animals Don't Get Heart Attacks – But People Do!* M R Publishing, 2000; see also Day, Phillip, *Health Wars*, ibid; Enstrom, J E, Kanim, L E & Klein, M A, "Vitamin C intake and Mortality", *Epidemiology 3*: pp.194-202; Willis G C, Light A W & W S Gow, "Serial Arteriography in Atherosclerosis", *Canadian Medical Association Journal* (1954) 71: pp.562-568; Ginter E, "Vitamin C Deficiency Cholesterol Metabolism and Atherosclerosis", *Journal of Orthomolecular Medicine* (1991) 6:pp.166-173; Ginter, E, "Marginal Vitamin C Deficiency, Lipid Metabolism and Atherosclerosis" *Lipid Research* 16: pp.216-220, 1978

dentist, chocolate! If we don't have magnesium in our soil, the crops won't have it either.

A comparison of data on food from 1930 and 1980, published in the British Food Journal in 1997, compared twenty vegetables and found levels of calcium, iron and other minerals had declined significantly. While our growers have concentrated on food that looks good, the emphasis has not been on mineral content. And whilst we are telling people to modify their diets, reduce fat and eat more fruit and vegetables, are we actually receiving the mineral requirements for good health? In many areas, we have empty foods unable to equip the body with the cellular nutrition required to build healthy cells capable of combating different stressors.

MERCURY AND DENTAL AMALGAMS
In the dental arena, the battle still rages over the use of the mercury-based amalgam fillings. Mercury is one of the most toxic materials known to man, and yet it is in our fillings. According to the University of Tennessee Toxicology Center Poisons Grading Unit, plutonium is graded at 1900, while mercury stands at 1600 and nickel at 600. Dental amalgam fillings contain about 50% mercury.

Since the beginning of the 20th century, amalgam has been widely accepted as a cost-effective and convenient filling material for teeth. There was concern when it was first used and there is concern again that it can cause long-term health problems for some patients. So this chemical stressor sits in the teeth 24 hours a day, seven days a week, 52 weeks a year, releasing mercury into the body. Cancer today now affects one person in three in most industrialised nations. What of multiple sclerosis and other neurological disorders that are also on the increase? Mercury is a neurotoxin.

FLUORIDE COMPOUNDS
Fluoride compounds found in our toothpastes, mouthwashes and some water supplies are alleged to reduce tooth decay. They are listed by the US Agency for Toxic Substances and Disease Registry (ATSDR) to be among the top 20 of 275 substances that pose the most significant threat to human health. Yet we use them twice a

day and dentists around the world recommend fluoride additives unabashedly. What's going on here?[18]

The New Jersey Department of Health reported osteosarcoma (bone cancer) rates were between three and seven times higher in fluoridated areas than in non-fluoridated areas.[19] Now we have tooth decay, dental fluorosis, hip fractures and osteosarcoma. Not bad for an additive used to reduce tooth decay in children![20] Here we are, placing toxic substances into the mouth with its wonderful transmucosal delivery system, and we're wondering why the world is getting sick.

These accumulating chemical stressors are causing real damage to the body. Yet there is a great deal of toothpaste used by millions of people with millions of dental amalgams stuck in their heads – people who don't appear to be sick. Dr Weston Price has this to say:

"Dental infections, while potentially harmful, may not be causing apparent or serious injury until the individual is subjected to some other overload, at which time a serious break may come. The chief contributing overloads are influenza, pregnancy, lactation, malnutrition, exposure, grief, worry, fear and age." [21]

To Dr Price's list can be added dental chemical stressors such as mercury, sodium fluoride and hexafluorosilicic acid - the raw toxic waste added to drinking water supplies, apparently to prevent dental decay.

On a daily basis, the body is being exposed to a vast array of stressors, toxins, pollutants and the rigors of everyday life. Selye states that the effects of these stressors are cumulative. Disease

---

[18] Maurer et al, *Journal of the National Cancer Institute*, Vol. 82, 1990, pp.1118-26; also Valerian, Val, "On The Toxic Nature of Fluorides", *Perceptions*, October 1995

[19] Valerian, Val, *Perceptions*, ibid.

[20] *Journal of the American Medical Association*, 3/8/95, 8/11-12/92, 7/25/91, 6/19/91, 7/25/90; *American Journal of Epidemiology*, 4/91; *American Journal of Public Health*, 7/90

[21] Price, Weston A, *Nutrition and Physical Degeneration*, Price-Pottenger Nutrition Foundation, La Mesa, California, 1979

isn't an overnight experience, but one where a slow, progressive assault on the body eventually causes a state of 'disease' to become known.

STOP PAYING HIM

Yet we still wait until we're sick before we seek help. With all due respect to the medical profession, which treats people once they have the problem, we need to take care of ourselves so that the problems do not originate in the first place. Contrast the Chinese system with our own. They pay the doctor all the while they are well, but *stop paying him* when they're sick. We wait until we're sick, and then suffer the hefty medical bills. Admittedly, under socialised healthcare, it doesn't appear to cost us anything, except that, in Britain's case, the citizen bears one of the highest taxation burdens in the world. And then there are the National Health Service waiting lists. By the time your turn comes, an illness will have often progressed to a dangerous condition which absolutely would not have been the case with early intervention.

SICK, NOT SICK

The plain fact is that just because we are not clinically sick, that does not mean that we are well. Have you ever felt this way? Sick and tired of feeling sick and tired. You go off to the doctor who checks you out and finds nothing wrong. All the tests come back negative and you get a clean bill of health. You still feel sick and tired, but you can't be - the doctor says you're okay! Let's change this around slightly. There are two extremes: sick and well. Between them are 'not sick' and 'not well'. 'Sick, not sick' is what the doctor is there for. 'Well, not well' is very probably our own responsibility.

SYMPTOM-BASED MEDICATION

In the state of 'sick, not sick', watch what happens: you are going nowhere with your health, since the treatment you receive from your doctor is to keep you 'not sick'. This treatment is almost always symptom-based medication that attempts to keep the symptoms at bay but won't make you better. This is almost always the effect of psychiatric drugs – medications that do not correct the underlying causes of mental illness, but merely suppress the symptoms of the illness, rendering the patient more acceptable to friends, family and society.

BLOOD THINNERS

A lady came to see me recently for a dental check-up. She had been putting this off as the doctor had put her on the blood-thinning drug, Warfarin. She was concerned that I might make her bleed. Her friends had told her that dentists don't like treating people on blood thinners. Actually, this is not true. But we do have to take precautions if we are going to extract a tooth. This lady's Warfarin was for an irregular heartbeat, to prevent the possibility of heart attack, stroke, pulmonary embolism and deep-vein thrombosis. She had witnessed the deaths of five of her close friends and relatives. The final straw was the tragic death of her mother.

Within three days of the last death, she began suffering palpitations and irregular heartbeats. Consultation with her doctor confirmed that she had a heart problem and the prescription was duly issued. She now awaits a specialist appointment. On discussion with the doctor, I said, *"So this is it? She's crossed the line and will be on medication for the rest of her life? No cure, just making sure that we keep her alive for as long as possible?" "Yes,"* he agreed. *"Basically that's the situation."*

This is 'sick, not sick'! This is what Selye called the stage of exhaustion that ultimately ends in death.

WELL, NOT WELL

What happened to 'well, not well'? The Chinese believe in the power of regeneration through good nutrition and Chinese medicine. Whilst there are some rather questionable aspects to some of the theory behind Chinese or Eastern Medicine, an understanding of the concept of nutrition is key in our journey to health.

While we cannot change our environment totally for the better, we can change our personal situation. Why take the risk of using toxic substances on and in the body when there are safe alternatives? Why accept the idea that we all die of ill-health when the goal should be to die WELL? They do so in at least 18 cultures across the world today – and at grand old ages too![22]

HARMLESS ALTERNATIVES

In this book we look at what is out there that will harm you and suggest some excellent, safe alternatives. If you are going to use toothpaste or have a filling, then does it not make sense to go for the harmless? Why take an unnecessary gamble with your health? If you're looking to be well, you need to reduce the harmful stressors that have the potential to make you sick.

For too long, we have assumed that if we buy it from the supermarket, it's safe. **This is absolutely not the case**. Many products have been 'grandfathered' into the public domain, with no government testing or approval <u>and no formal regulation</u>. Hard to believe? Read on!

---

[22] Day, Phillip, *Health Wars*, Credence, 2001

Sweet Temptation

I could feel the pain in her voice. There was no mistaking it. She had hung on all night, hoped to make it through to Monday. But now the pain was so intense, she could hardly speak. Her voice quivered as she told me how this sharp, excruciating pain shot up through her tooth and filled her whole head with agony - a pain so intense that no painkiller touched it. Sleep was out of the question, the hand on the clock just dragged itself around the dial. All she could do was sit and rock from side to side, waiting for the morning and the hope that her dentist would come out and see her on a Sunday.

The tooth is proud in the mouth but mobile, raised by the sea of pus swimming around its roots. This is pain, excruciating pain, sleepless pain, suicide pain. A local anaesthetic takes the edge off and then the relief as the drill opens up the tooth and the pressure of pus explodes up the root canal to dissipate into the aspirator. With the pain gone, a weak smile can be raised and the patient is off home to bed. A night never to be repeated.

And yet this agony goes on all over the world, day and night, year in, year out. Maybe your turn, maybe your child's. Toothache! There's nothing quite like it!

Nobody wants it. So why do we set ourselves up to get it?

THE KILLING FIELDS
"Sugar and spice and all things nice",
"Sweets for my sweet, sugar for my honey",
"My boy lollipop, oh no! no! no!"

We sing about it, laugh about it, sell it to our kids, and call it a treat. If you're good, you'll get a sweet. The first prize is a box of candy, a party bag. Of course, you've already eaten birthday cake laden with sugar icing covered with little colourful chocolate drops. You've tucked into jelly and trifle, washed down with sugar water masquerading as lemonade. Why not go home with your energy bag of goodies, decay on a stick, pain in a wrapper, and red colouring, to ensure that by the time you reach mum and dad, you are hyper, out of control, angry and tearful, with sleep never the option.

SEARING PAIN

When tiredness finally overcomes your frail body, you fall into a restless sleep, only to be woken at three in the morning with that sharp, lancing, searing pain shooting up through your tooth, exploding into your brain. The cycle begins again. Working in the dental emergency department gives real insight into this problem, repeated over and over again. Different faces, different homes, different backgrounds, yet all with same problem: dental pain caused by the ravages of tooth decay. All this from the innocent sugar cane standing so tall in the fields, swaying in the breeze, waiting to be harvested, refined and sprinkled on your cornflakes.

WHO PAYS?

"What kind of fool am I?" The kind that believes it won't harm me? Yet I do it again and again. Even after I say I'll never do it again - I do it again.

And what of the parent, who says of his four-year-old, *"I told her, if she ate sweets, her teeth would go rotten"*? Right. Like your four-year-old goes out to work, earns money and then disappears off to the sweet shop with the full knowledge of what she is doing and the understanding that a high intake of refined sugar will be responsible for a pH change in her oral environment, for the breakdown of dental enamel and the onset of tooth decay! I don't think so.

WHITE FLOUR - THE CULPRIT

In his book on nutrition and physical degeneration, Weston Price cites the Western diet of highly refined sugar and white flour as the culprits, causing dental decay and the crowding of the teeth with narrowing of the dental arches and the onset of modern disease in tribes who had previously lived on a 'primitive' diet.[23] Primitive? Maybe they were better off before we got to them.

---

[23] Price, Weston, A, *Nutrition and Physical Degeneration*, ibid.

SWEET DECAY

Am I blaming sucrose? Yes! Does it actually cause disease? You'd better believe it. *"But it gives me energy!"* I hear you say. *"My children won't eat their breakfast cereal without it! And coffee without sugar? I might as well not drink it!"* So don't. We'll come on to caffeine a little later.

CHOICE

Life is about choice. Am I really saying that you can't enjoy yourself, indulge at your favourite restaurant, load up on your strawberries with all those pretty white granules and suck on those after-dinner mints? Yes, I am. It's my job to say these things. After all, I am a dentist! But if you all give up sugar, the dentist's Porsche will have to go back. No more private education for the kids, or holidays on the Barrier Reef. So go ahead, make my day. Chew on! (Actually I drive around in a beaten-up old Volvo and indulge in no exotic holidays - more's the pity.)

AVOIDING SUGAR IS CRUCIAL

Dental researcher Professor Brian Burt, BDS, at the University of Michigan, reported to a National Institutes of Health panel in March 2001: *"...Avoiding consumption of excess sugar is a justifiable part of caries prevention, if not the most crucial aspect."*[24]

"We are wasting taxpayers' money researching fluoride, when it's clear that improper diet leads to tooth decay." says lawyer Paul Beeber, President of the New York State Coalition Opposed to Fluoride. *"Sadly, it is fluoride's adverse effects that hurt and malnourish the most, including neurological impairment, bone deformities, dental defects, thyroid dysfunction and more."* [25]

TRUTH DECAY

It has long been accepted that sugar plays an important role in tooth decay. Yet, according to the United States Food and Drug Administration (FDA), the average person still consumed 40

---

[24] NYS Coalition Opposed to Fluoridation, New York, 2nd May, 2001
[25] NYS Coalition Opposed to Fluoridation, ibid.

pounds of sugar in 1985. This is an average of 12 teaspoons a day. According to Nancy Appleton Ph.D. this is grossly inaccurate.[26] The University of California Berkeley Wellness letter reported the largest sugar consumption at 133 pounds of sugar per person per year. In 1986 the FDA came out with a report concerning the consumption of sugar in the United States and its possible effects on health. It reported that when the consumption of sugar reached 20 to 25% of a person's diet, people began to develop medical problems such as:

"Diabetes mellitus, glucose intolerance, cardiovascular risk, behavioural changes, gallstones and mineral deficiencies."[27]

The FDA concluded that, as the average American did not consume enough sugar to cause degenerative disease, the only risk from the sugar intake was tooth decay.

According to her report, Dr Appleton shows that the FDA miscalculated the intake of sugar. The 133 pounds of sugar eaten per year is a problem for many people and can lead to degenerative diseases. Our education has been to reduce sugar intake to prevent dental caries. While this is an important consideration, it would appear that sugar is far worse for us than just tooth decay, if eaten in large amounts.

The United States Department of Agriculture (USDA) estimates that in 1996, about 67 pounds of sugar (cane and beet), 85 pounds of corn sweeteners and 1 pound of other sweeteners (honey, maple syrup, etc.) per capita was delivered into the food supply. That adds up to a total nutritive sweetener of about 153 pounds per capita.[28] This figure is much nearer Dr Appleton's estimate and raises definite health questions. It is interesting that these figures appear to be paraded proudly by the sugar industry!

[26]Appleton, Nancy, "Where Has All The Sugar Gone?"
www.howtolearn.com/sugararticle.html
[27] Appleton, Nancy, ibid.
[28] *About Sugar: How much sugar do we eat?*
http://www.sugar.org/ scoop/aboutsug.html

SUCROSE

Dr William Coda Martin was the first person publicly to label sucrose a poison. Martin's definition came about after he determined the classical definition of a poison was *"...any substance applied to the body, which causes or may cause disease."*[29] The dental profession is still unsure as to the exact cause of tooth decay. Theories abound that sugar is the culprit. *Streptococcus mutans*, in conjunction with sucrose in the oral cavity, is the most potent caries-inducing infectious agent in the body. It is generally agreed that bacteria attach themselves to dental plaque formed on the tooth surface. The bacterial breakdown causes an acid to be released, which eats away the tooth enamel. Weston Price conducted thousands of experiments to determine the reasons for tooth decay.

POLITICAL AGENDA

For political reasons Price's conclusions were hidden for years. He discovered from patient blood analysis that the acid-base balance of the body in dental infections changed from its normal, slightly alkaline status to acidic. Harold Hawkins D.D.S. demonstrated that the saliva of people free of dental decay was alkaline, while that of those suffering dental decay was acidic. Hawkins states that this acidity...

"...is due to a diet rich in white bread, cereal, cookies, cake, sugar and other refined foods." [30]

ROOT FILLINGS

Dr Price found that people who had root fillings and tooth decay also had a lowered ionic calcium level in both the blood and saliva. Thus, it would appear from Price's work that dental decay is a whole-body event. It is systemic rather than just a localised reaction. The need to modify that sugary diet is therefore much more important than just reducing dental decay. It plays a major role in the reduction of degenerative diseases. Phillip Day again:

---

[29] Martin, William Coda, "When is a Food a Food – and When a Poison?" *Michigan Organic News*, March, 1957, p.3
[30] Meinig, George, *Root Canal Cover-up*, Bion Publishing, 1994

"Britain has had two things working against her from the start, not suffered by other countries around the world. She was the first industrialised nation. Suddenly, a tremendous shift in production went from the land and agriculture into the cities.

In the 1800's, Britain became a world empire, controlling over a quarter of the globe – her unlikely rise to power due to her army and navy, her massive new industrial output and ingenious innovation. Britain became the world centre for commercially produced sugar, biscuits and confectionery and the burgeoning companies overseeing this tremendous output were ever keen on the bottom line.

Their work forces were fed the cheap, easily available diets predominant in the products they produced: lard, sugar, refined white bread and flour and salted meat. By the end of the 1800s, the health of the working class had been ruined, cancer and heart disease were on the up, and the condition and smell of rotting British teeth were making the Empire's camels wince as far away as Baghdad.

By the 1930's, it was well known in scientific circles that bad food, lacking freshness and nutrients, was the major cause of wrecked health among the working classes in Britain. And of course, Britain exported its errant diet to those nations within its sphere of control."[31]

RAMPANT DECAY

In children, rampant dental caries is still seen today. It is rampant because many tooth surfaces are attacked by the decay process. Often you will see children with brown, broken, decaying front teeth. Mum has used a pacifier with a bit of sugar or honey on it or a feeding bottle with the teat filled with a sugary drink to settle the child at night. The decay is slow, no real pain; sometimes a bit of sensitivity and then they appear in the surgery or the emergency clinic with intense pain, usually late at night. Because they can't sleep, they're fractious, irritable, tired and the throbbing pain only makes things worse. This is not a good time to be a dentist. Bottle

---

[31] Day, Phillip, *Health Wars*, ibid.

or pacifier decay tends to be found at the front of the mouth. Sugary foods tend to attack the rest of the teeth as well.

THE WRONG CONCLUSION

A study of children in Manchester found that two in five of all three year-olds had some dental decay, while in neighbouring, poorer Salford, nearly half were affected. The Greater Manchester survey of 762 three year-olds found that in Manchester itself, 40% of people had some dental decay. One in five had serious decay, with the whole enamel layer broken down. Dr Gill Hawley, the senior dental officer at Mancunian Community Healthcare NHS Trust who carried out the survey, declared: *"Sugary drinks were the number one culprit."* [32]

CONFUSED CONCLUSION

A spokesman for the British Dental Association (BDA) said:

"The figures aren't surprising. They reinforce what we already know: that children in socially deprived areas, who don't have fluoride, are likely to have the worst decay rates." [33]

Whoa!! Did I really read this? Interesting conclusion. Since it was already stated that sugar was the number one culprit, the cause, the assailant, tell me how we got this jump to fluoride? Let's back up here for a minute. If the causative agent is sugar, then surely, even in a deprived area, we need to reduce the sugar intake? What has this got to do with fluoride supplementation?

It is well known that in socially deprived areas tooth decay is higher. What is interesting is the BDA stance on fluoride. It endorses the use of water fluoridation, suggesting that fluoride will help bring tooth decay under control. Later in the book, we will look at fluoride where some interesting facts, contrary to the BDA opinion, will be raised.

---

[32] BBC News, "Tooth Decay Rampant Among Toddlers"
http://news.bbc.co.uk/hi/english/health/newsid_368000/368803.stm
[33] BBC News, "Tooth Decay Rampant Among Toddlers", ibid.

COLA-MAN

I saw a young lad this week with a hole in his front tooth. Nothing incredible about that. It was his attitude that amazed me. Here was an intelligent young man from a good family who thought it funny that he could consume ten to fifteen cans of cola in a day. When I suggested he stop, I might just as well have drowned him in his cola, so great was his need for this drink. The only outward, visible effect was the hole on the front surface of his upper left lateral incisor... so far. What will happen to him in the years to come if he continues this practice?

PURE?

Once again, sugary drinks are implicated. Parents attempting to reduce tooth decay have turned away from the so-called high-sugar drinks to the 'pure' fruit juices. When used in a bottle or feeding cup, these can still have devastating results. I had a family of health-minded patients who gave their sons diluted, pure apple juice. All three boys suffered tooth decay.

RIBENA COURT CASE

GlaxoSmithKline, which manufactures Ribena Toothkind, a blackcurrant soft drink, went to the UK High Court after its advertising campaign for the product fell foul of the Advertising Standards Authority.[34] The company stated that its special formula with added calcium counters the impact of fruit acids on the teeth and minimises erosion. The ASA ruled that the campaign was misleading and that GSK's claims that the drink did not encourage tooth decay should be removed from the packaging. The ASA claimed that the drink was less harmful than other sugary drinks, rather than not harmful at all. This product was accredited by the British Dental Association. The judge stated:

> "All the evidence now before me is to the effect that Ribena Toothkind does not produce the potential for tooth decay to any significant degree." But, he added: "Even 'negligible risk' and 'no substantial risk' must not be classed as 'no risk'."

---

[34] BBC News," Glaxo in Ribena High Court Hearing"
http://news.bbc.co.uk/hi/english/health/newsid_1121000/1121749.stm

WHICH ON THE CASE

Consumer magazine *Which* found that there were still high levels of sugar in the drink, although not as high as some other drinks aimed at children. The company cites 1,200 pages of scientific data to substantiate the claim that the drink does not encourage tooth decay. They have just received another three-year accreditation by the British Dental Association.

Since then, sugar has been named as one of the major players in tooth decay. Any sugar, even reduced sugar, will cause tooth erosion. The difficulty arises from the idea that reduced sugar is harmless. This encourages us to believe that we can drink more of it and all will be okay. The BDA actually recommends water or milk as the favourable drink for children. So why do parents go for the sweet drink? Because it pacifies the child until tooth decay sets in. Then there's the uphill battle, dealing with a difficult child in pain.

HYPER-KIDS – ATTENTION DEFICIT DISORDER

Sugar not only affects the teeth but moods too. According to Dr Allen Buresz:

"The vast majority of medical doctors consider Attention Deficit Disorder (ADD) to be of unknown causes. Yet it is a known fact that the elimination of food additives and refined sugar produces dramatic improvements. Surely it would be wiser to remove these products from the child's diet than to subject them to the widespread and indiscriminate use of drugs, especially Ritalin, for quick, short-cut suppression of deeper problems?" [35]

Hyperactivity has been diagnosed for hundreds of years, yet it has apparently become massively more prevalent in recent times due to the increased use of chemicals, pollutants, or heavy metal toxicity, such as lead, mercury, and cadmium. Medicine's answer to the problem has predictably revolved around the use of drugs such as Ritalin to solve the problems. In 1996, the World Health Organisation warned that Ritalin overuse had reached dangerous proportions.

---

[35] Buresz, Allen, "Attention Deficit Disorder & Hyperactivity Success" http://www.all-natural.com/add.html

While the American Dental Association refutes the validity of mercury poisoning as a cause of ADD, autism and Alzheimer's, leading mercury scientist Dr Haley disagrees. He states that:

"Mercury is a well-known, potent neurotoxin, and common sense would lead to the conclusion that severe neurotoxins would exacerbate all neurological disorders, including Parkinson's, ALS, MS, autism and ADD." [36]

According to Dr Haley, there are several research papers in refereed, high-quality journals and scientific publications which have shown how mercury inhibits the same enzymes in normal brain tissues that are inhibited in ADD brain samples.

NEUROTRANSMITTERS

In treating this condition, sugar should be removed from the diet and the use of mercury stopped. In addition to this, DHA and the essential fatty acids Omega 3 and 6, which help to form the cell membrane and synaptic endings of neurons in the brain and nervous system, should be used. All the important neurotransmitters are manufactured by the body from dietary sources. This means that the diet needs to be rich in the essential fatty acids consumed in the right ratio. In order for these neurotransmitters to work well, the B vitamins, magnesium, zinc, and Vitamin C must all be present in sufficient amounts. An effective ionised liquid trace mineral and vitamin supplement, together with an antioxidant and essential fatty acid supplement, would form a good baseline for the treatment of this condition. (See chapter on nutrition). Researcher Dr Joseph Mercola remarks:

"Another reason to avoid sugar is to slow down the ageing process. If you want to stay looking young, it is very important to limit sugar to the smallest amount possible. It is the most significant factor that accelerates ageing. It is a negative fountain of youth. It does this by attaching itself to proteins in the body, forming new sugar-protein substances called advanced glycation

---

[36] Haley, B, "Leading Mercury Scientist Refutes ADA in Congressional Testimony", www.mercola.com

35

end-products. The higher the AGE levels, the faster you are ageing. Sugar also increases oxidation elements in the body [described in current theory as free radicals] *which accelerate the ageing process.*"[37]

DEVOID OF NUTRITIONAL VALUE

Refined sugar is manufactured from cane and beet extract, which is emptied of its salts, proteins, vitamins and minerals. This leaves a white crystalline substance devoid of any nutritional value. In foods, sugar has been called carbohydrate. This allows the manufacturer to use sugar without telling you exactly how much you're getting. Labelling sugar a 'carbohydrate' means that the manufacturer can conceal the real content of sugar in the product.

TOXIC METABOLITES

Simple sugars such as fructose found in fruits are easily metabolised by the body into glucose, the only fuel your brain will use. They have the essential minerals and vitamins to enable fructose to be converted to glucose, used by the body for energy. Sucrose is devoid of these vitamins and minerals and cannot be completely digested by our bodies with the result that toxic metabolites are formed. In a short time, the blood sugar level drops and that sense of wellbeing descends into sluggishness. Sugar! We love it, but it's a slow poison.

Weston Price found that primitive tribes fed on white flour and sugar went from being fit, healthy people to tribes suffering the same degenerative diseases as so-called 'modern man'. His studies of the people in the Swiss Alps, Eskimos and primitive isolated Canadian Indians, Australian Aborigines, African tribes, Peruvian Indians, Torres Strait Islanders and isolated Polynesians all documented this sorry fact.

Our less-than-nourishing 'civilised' diet not only ravaged these sturdy peoples' teeth and physiques, but moral decay and criminal tendencies surfaced once the body and unfed brain became affected.

---

[37] "Reversing Damage Caused by Sugar to Fight Ageing", Issue 159, 2000 www.mercola.com

GREATEST HAZARDS

So we can look at our society today and reflect on the work of Dr Price. We can draw our own conclusions as we look at the work of C L Burt on delinquent and backward children whom he found to be frail, sickly and infirm. And we can look at our own people, crime rates, decline in morality and an increase in degenerative illnesses. Sugar drinks, fast foods and sugar-filled canned foods are one of the greatest hazards to man.

SUGAR DAMAGES ARTERIES

A new study from the University of Buffalo suggests that sugar may also be bad for your blood vessels and many other parts of the body. [38] The study showed:

- Excess sugar in the bloodstream stimulates free-radical production.
- Increases in incidences of type 2 diabetes occur with free-radical generation.
- Weight loss reduces free-radical production (earlier research).

They gave 14 healthy men and women, who had fasted for 12 hours, a drink composed of 75 grams of glucose - roughly equivalent to the sugar content of two cans of soda. 6 control patients drank a water-saccharin solution.

In subjects who drank the sugar water, free-radical generation increased significantly, while there was no change in the control group. Levels of alpha-tocopherol (Vitamin E) - a powerful antioxidant, fell by 4% after hour two and remained depressed after hour three.

A SPOONFUL OF SUGAR

So here we have it: we're sitting down to tea and cakes, all the while speeding up the ageing process; all the expense is on creams,

---

[38] "Sugar Creates Free Radicals and Reduces Vitamin E Levels"
www.mercola.com/2000/aug/27/sugar_free_radicals.htm

pills and potions, when it would appear that all it takes is to cut out those helpings of sugar!

SACCHARIN - A SWEET ALTERNATIVE OR A CARCINOGEN?

What's the alternative? Over the years, the food industry has been looking at alternative ways to feed our craving for all things sweet - a commendable project and, while one would expect to see a reduction in tooth decay, other problems make those sweeteners a less than viable alternative.

"Saccharin is a carcinogen. Do not use it," declares leading toxicologist, Samuel Epstein MD. [39]

Three important studies showed saccharin caused an increase in bladder cancer in rats: the Wisconsin Alumni Research Foundation in 1973, the FDA in 1973 and Arnold *et al* from Canada's Health Protection Branch. These studies confirmed that saccharin induced bladder, uterine and ovarian cancer. [40]

In 1977, British medical journal The Lancet published a paper entitled *"Artificial Sweeteners and Human Bladder Cancer."* Written under the auspices of the Canadian National Cancer Institute, it was found that there was a 65% greater risk of developing bladder cancer in those who used saccharin than those who didn't. It was also found that the risk increased over time.

BLADDER TUMOURS

Dr Elizabeth M Whelan explains some of the problems related to saccharin:

"Saccharin, which has been used as an alternative to sugar since the early 20th century, officially assumed the 'carcinogen' title in March 1977, when a rodent study in Canada produced an excess of bladder tumours in male animals." [41]

---

[39] Steinman, D & Epstein, S S *The Safe Shopper's Bible*, Macmillan, 1995

[40] Epstein, Samuel S, *The Politics of Cancer Revisited*, East Ridge Press, USA, www.preventcancer.com

[41] Whelan, Elizabeth M, "The Sweet and the Sour News about Saccharin", American Council on Science and Health, 17th May 2000

This finding immediately triggered the threat of the so-called 'Delaney Clause' - a congressionally mandated provision that requires the Food & Drug Administration to ban literally 'at the drop of a rat' any synthetic food chemical shown to cause cancer when ingested by laboratory animals.

WEIGHT OF OPINION
When millions of weight-conscious Americans heard that their only available low-calorie sweetener was going to be banned (cyclamates had been banned in 1970 for similar reasons), they were outraged – and immediately bought up every little pink packet they could find. Congress responded to this outrage by protecting saccharin from the Delaney Clause and allowing it back on the market with a health-warning label. Saccharin's reputation was further tarnished when the US National Toxicology Program, referring again to the Canadian rat study, elected to put saccharin on its 'cancer-causing' list - formally declaring it 'an anticipated human carcinogen'. [42]

SACCHARIN - A CAUSE OF WEIGHT GAIN!
As part of a weight-loss program, saccharin also falls short of the mark. It was found in 1947 that as little as 50mg of saccharin would lower the blood sugar by 16%. As hunger is triggered by lowered blood sugar, the net effect induces the person to eat more. Neither is there any evidence that saccharin is helpful in diabetes.

Saccharin is used in toothpaste as a sweetener. In his book, *The Politics of Cancer Revisited,* Dr Epstein points out that saccharin is currently approved by the FDA as an intentional food additive. The current food additive law requires proof of safety and function, but not of efficacy or benefit. This means that an additive must perform its registered function.

A CASE OF SEMANTICS
For instance, a sweetener must sweeten food or a colour must colour food, but this function does not necessarily have to serve any useful purpose. In toothpaste, it serves the function of making it

---

[42] Whelan, Elizabeth M, "The Sweet and Sour News about Saccharin", ibid.

taste good. It could be argued that if toothpaste is not ingested, it surely can cause no harm. We will see later, when studying the fluoride debate, that toothpaste is ingested. In some countries like the USA, notice is given in writing on toothpaste cartons and tubes that if toothpaste is swallowed, the individual should seek immediate medical advice or contact a poisons control centre immediately!

ASPARTAME

Aspartame was discovered by accident in 1965 by James Schlatter, a chemist working for G D Serle Company. Its use as a sweetener was initially blocked in August 1974 by neuroscientist John W Olney and consumer attorney James Turner, due to concerns about its safety. In 1983 however, aspartame received its approval as a sweetener for fizzy drinks, despite growing concerns over its neurological effects. Dr Fereydoon Batmanghelidj has this to say on aspartame:

"In the intestinal tract, aspartame converts to two highly excitatory neurotransmitter amino acids: aspartate and phenylalanine, as well as methyl alcohol/formaldehyde (wood alcohol). Aspartate converts GTP energy to stockpile GMP, a spent fuel that causes thirst and hunger in an attempt to replace the lost energy stockpiles in the brain. Thus, diet sodas cause indiscriminate overuse of the energy reserves of cells in the brain."[43]

This of course gives an effect quite contrary to the desired one of weight loss. The hunger makes you overeat when the body doesn't really need the food with a resultant weight gain rather than loss. What an evil cycle. The sales pitch is so great, that for many, fear rather than fact will keep them on the treadmill, hoping, believing, trusting that the manufacturer is telling the truth.

Possible side-effects of aspartame include multiple sclerosis, Alzheimer's disease, ALS, memory loss, hormonal problems,

---

[43] Batmanghelidj, F *Your Body's Many Cries for Water*, Tagman Press, 2001. (Available at www.credence.org)

hearing loss, epilepsy, Parkinson's disease, brain lesions and neuro-endocrine disorders.

NEUROSTRESSORS

Aspartame affects neurotransmitters. Mercury is a neurotoxin, as is aluminium. Could Selye have been right? Add one neurostressor to another; combine their effects, and what are the possibilities that you might lose major mental function?

Quick Silver - The Case of Mercury Quackery

Contrary to popular opinion, 'quick silver' was not the comment made by the Lone Ranger when he wanted his trotting four-legged friend to move up a gear and gallop off into the sunset. It's a poisonous silvery metallic element, atomic number 80, according to current chemistry theory - a liquid at ordinary temperatures, known as mercury. It is also used in thermometers and amalgam fillings.

There's a hole in my tooth, dear Lisa, dear Lisa...
With what shall we fill it?

Is a question that has been going on for over 150 years. A question that actually divided the American Society of Dental Surgeons in 1856. Mercury/silver paste was introduced as a filling material into America in the 1830's, having been used in England and France by the early 1800's and by the Chinese as far back as the 7th century.[44] Mercury was known to be a poison and as it was widely recognized that exposure to it resulted in overt side-effects that included dementia (hence: mad as a Hatter) and loss of motor coordination, the Society and affiliated groups drew up a pledge for its members to sign. This pledge banned the use of amalgam. Those practitioners who violated this pledge were suspended for malpractice.

MALPRACTICE PREVAILS
Undeterred by this pledge, the advocates of amalgam prevailed - a decision that caused not only the division but also the downfall of the American Society of Dental Surgeons. They found the filling material cheap, easy to use and effective. It replaced cement, gold, lead and tinfoil as an alternative that was cost-effective and within the financial means of the majority of the American population. Support for the idea gained acceptance and the club was formed. In

---

[44] Lorscheider, F, L, Vimy, M J, and Summers, A O, "Mercury Exposure From Silver Tooth Fillings: Emerging Evidence Questions a Traditional Dental Paradigm", *FASEB Journal*, 1995

1859, The American Dental Association was founded, based on the advocacy of amalgam as a safe and desirable tooth-filling material. This society is alive today and beating the same drum.

AMALGAM

Amalgam filling is 50% mercury combined with 35% silver, 9% tin, 6% copper and a trace of zinc; easy to use, cheap and effective. From a practitioner's point of view, you can't really fault the material on its ease of use. It's a forgiving medium, even when packed slightly high. As long as it doesn't break within the first twenty-four hours of use, it will wear down. You might get toothache from the high filling, and perhaps headaches, but these settle as the filling wears in. The dental profession is doing its job, filling decayed teeth with a cost-effective material that is durable and with financial appeal to a vast consumer market looking for the best deal they can get. Everybody is happy! So what's the problem?

MERCURY TOXIC? SURELY NOT!

There's one slight hitch, mercury is one the most toxic substances known to man.[45] The University of Tennessee has a renowned toxicology centre, where they grade poisons on the basis of the least amount necessary to kill a human being. As already covered, plutonium is the most deadly, and is rated on their scale at 1,900. Mercury stands at 1,600 and nickel 600. That's toxic. Organised dentistry has countered the controversy surrounding the toxicity of the mercury in dental fillings by claiming that it reacts with the other metals in the amalgam to form a 'biologically inactive substance', and by observing that dentists have not reported any adverse side-effects in their patients.

SAFETY NOT A CONSIDERATION

We dentists were taught that amalgam was a good filling material to use and that it was inert. According to the UK's National Health Service (NHS) Centre for Reviews and Dissemination (University of York), amalgam is the direct restorative material of

---

[45] Levenson, Jack, "Mercury Amalgams and Metal in the Mouth", http://www.mercury free.co.uk/mercury.html

choice, unless aesthetics are important.[46] There is no mention of toxicity. All we are told is just how good it is as a filling material. It's almost as if what happens in the body has nothing to do with the filling material. That there are serious questions over its safety never appears to be taken into consideration.

Dr. Dietrich Klinghardt, widely recognized as one of the most knowledgeable physicians on mercury detoxification, states:

"Chronic mercury exposure from occupational, environmental, dental amalgam and contaminated food exposure is a significant threat to public health. Those with amalgam fillings exceed all occupational exposure allowances of mercury exposure of all European and North American countries... People with an average of eight amalgam fillings could absorb up to 120 micrograms of mercury a day. These levels are consistent with reports of 60 micrograms of mercury collected from human faeces. By way of contrast, estimates of daily absorption of all forms of mercury from fish and seafood are 2.3 micrograms, with foods, air and water 0.3 micrograms per day."[47]

MERCURY ON THE BRAIN

The mercury vapour from amalgam fillings is lipid-soluble and passes readily through cell membranes and across the blood-brain barrier. One way the body rids itself of mercury is through the bile, which unfortunately empties into the intestine where it can be re-absorbed back into the bloodstream again.[48] Hence the link with neurological disease, Alzheimer's disease, neurotransmitter imbalances and multiple sclerosis. Thyroid problems and an impaired immune system are also implicated. Dr Klinghardt backs up his paper with 124 of the best literature documents on mercury detoxification. However, the British Dental Association fact file summarizes current thinking on the use of dental amalgam thus:

---

[46] The University of York, NHS Centre for Reviews and Dissemination. *Effective Health Care*, Vol 5, No 2, 1999
[47] Klinghart Dietrich, *The British Journal of Clinical Nutrition and Environmental Medicines* Vol. 11, March 1998
[48] Stejskal, Jenny, "Beware of Metals: A possible Cause of Immunological Disorders". c/o Melisa Medica Foundation c/o Stejskal Akeryvagen 336, 183 35 Taby, Sweden

"To date, extensive research has failed to establish any links between amalgam and ill-health. Those countries which are limiting the use of amalgam are doing so to lower environmental mercury levels." [49]

REFILLING KEEPS DENTISTS IN BUSINESS

Tooth decay is one of the most common diseases and accounts for almost half of all tooth extractions. The treatment of tooth decay by placement of simple, direct fillings costs the British National Health Service (NHS) £173 million per year (around US$248 million). While they may last a long time, these fillings are far from permanent, with over 60% of all restorative dentistry being for the replacement of restorations already performed. For the most part, these fillings are dental amalgams. They are not permanent but do, according to review, last the longest.

The more exposure to the filling material, the more chance that the body will become sensitive to it. It is believed that allergy to amalgam is estimated to be less than 1%. [50] A search of the scientific studies reveals however that as much as 16% of the population may be allergic to mercury. [51] Here we have a material that may be poisonous, is not permanent, can cause allergies, and yet is still the filling material of choice. Does this make sense? What are we in the dental profession trying to defend? To be fair and accurate, not all dentists agree with the use of mercury-based amalgams. Many feel that the adverse reactions of the body to mercury amalgam make this material less than desirable as a filling medium.

IMMUNE SYSTEM CHALLENGED

In her paper on metals and immunological disorders, Jenny Stejskal points out that:

"Heavy metals in the body challenge the immune system. Since metals are substances foreign to the body, any abnormally

---

[49] BDA Fact file, *Dental Amalgam Safety*, January 1977
[50] Mitchell, E, NIDR/ADA Workshop on Biocompatibility of Metals in Dentistry, 11-13th July, 1984
[51] Nebenfurer, L et al, "Mercury Allergy in Budapest", *Contact Dermatitis* 10(2): 121-22 1983

high concentration of heavy metals will stimulate phagocytosis by macrophages and monocytes in order to protect the organism. These scavenger cells do not have the enzymes to metabolise the metals and so, on death of the cells, the metals are released back into the system. The metals preferably bind to tissues and organelles rich in sulphyl-groups, such as mitochondria. This may block or inhibit vital cell respiration. As a result, the cells may divide uncontrollably. By definition, this is the beginning of carcinogenesis.[52]

In 1984, a group of dentists formed the International Academy of Oral Medicine and Toxicology (IAOMT). Their objective was scientifically to explore the safety of amalgam restorations. Since this time, they have inspired many medical scientists at universities around the world to research possible patho-physiologic effects associated with mercury leaking from these restorations. Consequently, there are a growing number of scientific studies documenting patho-physiologic effects associated with amalgam mercury.

HOW THE TIDE HAS TURNED

Here we have the debate - a dental profession that is behind the use of amalgam as a safe material and the scientific world that disagrees. The dentists who agree with the scientists and refuse to use amalgam or replace it are called quacks (the derogatory word 'quack' may first have been used to describe someone using mercury preparations on the skin, deriving its name from 'quack salve'). How the tide has turned. Once the profession was against the use of mercury, now it is all for it. But does the evidence stack up in favour of this material or not?

According to IAOMT, it does not. There are fundamental health flaws to silver fillings that adversely affect a patient's health. Researchers have measured a daily release of mercury in the order of 10 micrograms from the amalgam into the body. This is not good. By scientific definition, mercury is a toxic metal - the most minute amounts will damage cells.[53]

---

[52] Stejskal, J, "Beware of Metals...", ibid.
[53] "Mercury-Free and Healthy - The Dental Amalgam Issue",

FILLINGS OR BATTERY?

The second fundamental flaw is that amalgam is made up of five dissimilar metals. Galvanic currents are inevitable. The electricity produced is between 0.1 and 10 micro-amps, compared to the body's natural current of 3 amps. Mercury leakage causes changes in the systems of the body that are often slow and insidious. This means that health problems may occur, years after amalgam placement.

The release of mercury from amalgams represents the primary source of mercury exposure in people with amalgam fillings. This release is six times the amount found in fish and seafood. Studies by the World Health Organization show that a single amalgam can release 3-17 mcg. of mercury a day, making amalgam a primary source of mercury exposure.[54]

TOXICITY BY INHALATION

A Danish study of a random sample of 100 men and 100 women showed that increased blood mercury levels were related to the presence of more than four amalgam fillings in the teeth. Since mercury vapour is released all the time, dental patients inhale mercury 24 hours a day, all year round. This release is in sufficient amounts to cause systemic disease.[55] This vapour is rapidly deposited and accumulates in the jaw area (causing gum disease), the gastrointestinal tract, liver, kidney and other organs and tissues.

SUPERBUGS

Research showed a statistically significant increase in the incidence of mercury-resistant bacteria during the five weeks following installation of amalgam fillings.[56] These findings indicate that mercury released from these fillings can cause an enrichment

---

http://www.amalgam.org

[54] www. alternativemedicine.com/digest/issue20/20700.shtml

[55] www.mercuryfree.co.uk

[56] Summers, A O, J Wireman, M J Vimy, F L Lorscheider, B Marshall, S B Levy, S Bennett, and L Billard, "Mercury released from dental silver fillings provokes an increase in mercury- and antibiotic- resistant bacteria in oral and intestinal floras of primates", *Antimicrobial Agents and Chemotherapy*, pp.825-834, April 1993

of mercury-resistant plasmids in the normal bacterial floras of primates. Many of these plasmids also carry antibiotic resistance, implicating the exposure to mercury from amalgam fillings in an increased incidence of multiple antibiotic plasmids.

Overuse of antibiotics in dentistry has been blamed for the increase in superbugs. It is therefore of interest to see that mercury is also implicated.

MAD DENTISTS

Dental personnel were researched with regard to neurological behavioural effects from dental amalgam mercury. The findings presented convincing new evidence of adverse behavioural effects associated with low mercury exposures.[57] According to Sandra Denton MD, dentists have the highest suicide and divorce rates among professionals. Female staff are more likely to abort. This is not a comforting thought for all those trusting nervous patients who look to their dentist and staff for stability.

Research has shown negative changes in haemoglobin levels, cellular energy production and white cell activity, all important in the function of our immune system as the latter combats infection, disease and cancer.[58] The cumulative evidence clearly shows that mercury has negative systemic health effects.

DANGER TO THE UNBORN CHILD

Mercury fillings have been linked to infertility[59], cardiac dysfunction[60], foetal development and Alzheimer's. It was once the case in Britain that while women were pregnant and eligible for free treatment under the terms of the NHS, they would have their

---

[57] Echeverria, D, H V Aposhian, J S Woods, N J Heyer, M M Aposhian, A C Bittner Jr, R K Mahurn and M Cianciola, "Neurobehavioural effects from exposure to dental amalgam Hg: new distinctions between recent exposure and Hg body burden", *FASEB Journal* 12, pp.971-980, 1998

[58] Adolph Coors Foundation, sponsored study, 1998

[59] Gerhard, I, Monga, B, Waldbrenner, A, Runnebaum, B, "Heavy metals and fertility", *Journal of Toxicology and Environmental Health*, Part A, 1998

[60] Frustaci, A et al Marked elevation of myocardial trace elements in ideopathic dilated cardiomyopathy compared with secondary cardiac dysfunction, *Journal Am. Coll. Cardiol*, 1999

48

amalgam fillings put in. However we have now been told not to undertake these fillings during pregnancy. This of course indicates that the authorities recognise the dangers to the developing foetus. If this is the case, one has to ask why we still use mercury and who sanctions it as a safe material anyway.

DENTIST OR FALL GUY?

There is some confusion here. According to Michael Ziff DDS, of the Foundation for Toxic-Free Dentistry in Orlando, Florida, the Food and Drug Administration (FDA) has never approved mixed dental amalgam. What they have done is to approve the two components that make up amalgam - mercury and dental alloy. Although charged by law to evaluate and classify every medical and dental device to be used on or in humans, the FDA has not evaluated or classified "mixed amalgam", the material used in 75-80% of all fillings. To avoid the issue, the FDA simply took the position that the amalgam was a reaction product manufactured by the dentist when the mercury and alloy were mixed prior to placement in the tooth.

In other words when you heard the click of the capsule and the whirr of the amalgamator, your dentist took over responsibility for the toxic material that was going to be placed in your tooth. This means that, as the practicing dentist, I have become the legal manufacturer of the end-product known as amalgam. I don't remember being told this at dental school!

In 1995 the following letter was sent out by the American Dental Association:

"The American Dental Association owes no legal duty of care to protect the public from allegedly dangerous products used by dentists. The ADA did not manufacture, design, supply or install the mercury-containing amalgams. The ADA does not control those who do. The ADA's only alleged involvement in the product was to provide information regarding its use. Dissemination of information relating to the practice of dentistry does not create a duty of care to protect the public from potential injury."

ARE DENTISTS RESPONSIBLE?

In a letter to the Federal President of the Australian Dental Association, Dr R Gammal, former President of the Australian Society of Oral Medicine and Toxicology, stated:

"It has come to my attention recently that in California a civil lawsuit has been filed by a person claiming that he sustained injuries by exposure to mercury in his dental amalgam fillings. He named as defendant his treating dentist, two amalgam manufacturers, an amalgam distributor and the American Dental Association. The ADA has eliminated itself from responsibility. Could you please comment?"[61]

The response of the Australian Dental Association on the 2nd August 1995 thanked Dr Gammal for his letter regarding the lawsuit, but was unaware of this situation. The author was surprised, quoting the "Hulet" case, where a practitioner's license had been revoked in California following his claims to cure various illnesses by removing amalgams.

The President of the ADA went on to say that: *"The position of the Association with regard to potential legal action was to seek the most expert advice in the matter. We do not pretend to be a scientific body with expertise in toxicology and systemic disease."*[62]

DO WE KNOW WHAT WE ARE DOING?

This would echo the view of the immuno-toxicologists who know that we don't have the knowledge to decide what should go into a tooth from a biocompatibility point of view. It is true; we study the sciences to gain entrance into dental school. We study dental materials but are also at the mercy of the scientists who manufacture the products that we use in the mouth.

So the debate goes full-circle. Who do you believe? The dentist, who is good at his job but, by his own admission, does not have the

---

[61] Gammal, R, President ASOMAT. Special newsletter announcement from the Australasian Society of Oral Medicine and Toxicology, September, 1995

[62] Dalton, P, Reply to Dr Gammal's letter printed in the same edition of the ASOMAT newsletter. Contact: http//www.asomat.com

scientific expertise to decide on the toxic effects of the filling materials that he uses? The American Dental Association, who wash their hands of all responsibility for the use of mercury fillings yet sanction their use? Or the body of scientific evidence that demonstrates amalgam fillings to be bad for you?

Mercury – The Current Position

According to IAOMT (International Academy of Oral Medicine and Toxicology), the governments of Austria, Finland, Germany and Sweden have already announced plans to limit the use of "dental mercury amalgams". The Canadian government has assented to place the amalgam issue under review by regulatory authorities. In 1997, an amalgam ban was demanded in Germany. This followed the largest study on mercury release from dental amalgams in the world. A translated press release by Matts Hanson, Ph.D. of Sweden, BUND, Friends of the Earth, The Association of Environment and Environmental Protection, Germany, demands: *"No respite for amalgam - amalgam ban overdue."*[63] The largest test in the world on mercury release from amalgam fillings into the saliva was initiated in summer 1995 by BUND and carried out by the Department of Environmental Analysis at the University of Tubingen. In the specially examined group of 21-40 year-old persons, the study established a statistically significant relationship between mercury levels in saliva and symptoms. The set of symptoms, often called 'micromercurialism' in the literature, were:

Mouth - oral cavity: bleeding gingiva, metal taste, burning tongue

Central nervous system: Concentration difficulties, impaired memory, sleep disturbances, lack of initiative, nervousness

Gastrointestinal tract: not specified

BUND demanded of the Minister of Health that he act immediately on the basis that:

- *Amalgam, as an additional risk factor, does not belong in the mouth.*
- *An amalgam ban should be not just for women and children, but the rest of the community.*

---

[63] *Bio-Probe News*, "Amalgam Ban Demanded by Germany." http://www.bioprobe.com/readNews.asp?article=11

- *University dental clinics should stop teaching amalgam use.*
- *Universities should teach their safe and proper removal.*[64]

A CASE FOR BRITISH UNDERSTATEMENT

On their web page for the public, the British Dental Association has a section for the public advising on the safety of filling materials. The Department of Health has advised dentists that amalgam fillings are free from risk of systemic toxicity - that they are not a threat to general health. The Department further states that very occasionally they can cause a local sensitivity reaction. Removal of the filling will end this. Apart from hypersensitivity, no health problems are thought to be caused by amalgam use, according to the British Government. The Department of Health has suggested that where clinically reasonable, the placement or removal of amalgam fillings is avoided in pregnancy. This advice was given as a precaution and not because of any evidence of harm to the baby's development or health.

MERCURY CONCENTRATES IN THE FOETUS

Vimy looked at maternal/foetal distribution of mercury released from dental amalgam fillings.[65] In a study carried out on pregnant sheep, he found that mercury from the amalgam fillings appeared in maternal and foetal blood and amniotic fluid within two days of filling placement. All tissues examined displayed mercury accumulation. In adults, the highest accumulation was found in the kidney and liver, whereas in the foetus, the highest amalgam mercury concentrations appeared in the liver and pituitary glands.

In the study, the placenta progressively concentrated mercury as gestation advanced to term, and milk concentration of amalgam mercury postpartum provides a potential source of mercury exposure to the newborn. While this sample was small, it does point

---

[64] *Bio-Probe News*, Amalgam Ban Demanded in Germany, ibid.

[65] Vimy, M J, Takahashi & Lorscheider, F L, "Maternal-foetal Distribution of Mercury (203 Hg) Released From Dental Amalgam Fillings", *American Journal of Physiology*, 1990

to a risk. Other studies including one on rats by Fredricksson et al, whose results indicate that prenatal exposure to mercury causes alteration to both spontaneous and learned behaviours, suggesting some deficit in adaptive functions.[66] So once again, we have a disagreement on whether mercury is safe for the unborn child.

WHAT WOULD YOU DO FOR YOUR FAMILY?

A good question to ask your dentist before he carries out treatment on you is whether he would have it done to himself or to one of his family. For example, I was on a course in 1998 where a retired professor of dentistry was asked whether he would have an NHS crown. He replied that he certainly would not!

Where do you go from here? What are your alternatives? If you don't have any amalgam fillings, you might consider using an alternative filling material if the thought of mercury-based fillings in your head bothers you.

If you already have amalgams, do you rush out to your local dentist for immediate removal of the offending fillings or not? Can you afford to do it? Do you want to? And for those of you who are dental-phobic, is it possible for you to undergo such treatment? What are the risks to you and your health and what symptoms might you display from exposure to these filling materials? These are the questions that you need to ask yourself. Does my dentist agree with amalgam replacement or is he an amalgam supporter? It's a minefield out there for each one of us as we pick our way through the maze of questions.

HEALTH CHECK

One way of simplifying this decision process is to do a health check. How do you feel? What are your symptoms today?

The following represents a summary of the symptoms of 1,569 patients in six different studies. It evaluates the health effects of replacing mercury-containing dental fillings with non-mercury

---

[66] Fredriksson, A et al, "Prenatal co-exposure to metallic mercury vapour and methyl mercury produce interactive behavioural changes in adult rats", *Neurotoxicol. Teratol.* 18(2): 129-34, 1996

alternatives. The data was derived from the following sources: 762 patient adverse reaction reports, submitted to the FDA by patients; 807 patient reports from Sweden, Denmark, Canada and the United States. Symptoms include:

Allergy
Anxiety
Bad temper
Bloating
Blood pressure problems
Chest pains
Depression
Dizziness
Fatigue
Intestinal problems
Gum problems
Headaches
Insomnia
Irregular heartbeat
Irritability
Lack of concentration
Lack of energy
Memory loss
Metallic taste
Multiple sclerosis
Muscle tremor

On elimination of mercury-containing dental fillings, this group showed an average improvement or cure of 84%.

Do any of these symptoms apply to you?

HISTAMINE
Multiple sclerosis is often sited as a problem of mercury toxicity. Dr Jonathan Wright's October 1999 issue of *Nutrition and Healing* is devoted entirely to MS. In this article, Dr Wright looks at the use of the natural amino acid derivative histamine in the treatment of MS. Histamine is a neurotransmitter derived from histadine. Histamine has been identified as a major cause of allergic reaction. Hence the use of antihistamines. However the

verbal report of 200 patients suffering with MS, who have used histamine treatment, showed a 72% improvement in symptoms. DeLack, an MS sufferer,[67] has been instrumental in developing a histamine combination named "Procarin." Procarin with a specialised dietary regime provides a great chance of making real improvements in symptoms. It might also be worth adding plenty of water to this regime.

BIOPROBE COMMENTS

Bioprobe.com commented that exposure to mercury vapour from dental amalgams could result in allergic reactions, as well as some inhibition of the immune system. In retrospective studies done by the amalgam patient support group in Sweden, there was about a 20% cure rate in those who had amalgam replacement. They wonder whether amalgam replacement might enhance the action of Procarin.

Research conducted at the University of Calgary Faculty of Medicine has demonstrated that trace amounts of mercury can cause the type of nerve damage characteristic of that found in Alzheimer's disease. The level of mercury exposure is consistent with those levels found in dental amalgam fillings. The scientist found that other metals, including aluminium, did not cause the damage.[68]

Professor H. Vasken Aposhian, Ph.D. questions whether we are taking unnecessary risk by using mercury. In a written submission to the Committee on Government Reform, he discusses mercury toxicity. Elemental mercury is the liquid silver found in dental fillings. At room temperature it vaporises. This mercury vapour is very toxic. Dental amalgams continuously emit toxic mercury vapour. Studies have shown that the greatest exposure of the American population to mercury is via dental amalgams.[69]

---

[67] Delack, E, EDMS, www.msviews.com
[68] Lorscheider, FL et al, "Retrograde Degeneration of Neurite Membrane Structural Integrity of Nerve Growth Following In-vitro Exposure to Mercury", *Neuroreport*, 12(4): 733-737. 2001
[69] Aposhian, H.V. Ph.D, Professor of Molecular and Cellular Biology, Professor of Pharmacology, University of Arizona. Tuscon, Arizona.

MERCURY CROSSES THE PLACENTA BARRIER

One should remember that mercury vapour can cross the placenta barrier and thus harm the developing central nervous system of the foetus.[70] The target organs for this vapour are the brain and kidney. Methyl mercury is in many kinds of fish, marine mammals and crustaceans. Those at risk are women of childbearing age, pregnant women, foetuses and very young children. Once in the system, it migrates to the brain where it is converted to mercuric mercury.

THE WHITE FILLING ALTERNATIVE

So if we can't use mercury based fillings, what can we use? Tooth-coloured dental restorative materials have gained popularity, for both non-amalgam dentists and patients who want their teeth to look good. This demand has given us two broad groups of materials. The composite resins and the glass ionomer cements. The composite resins consist of monomers together with high-loading, powdered inorganic fillers (basically plastic and finely ground, glass-like particles). A white light source acts as the catalyst to set this material. This is the nice blue light that glows in your mouth when you have one of these fillings placed. The result is a good-looking restoration with no mercury.

GLASS IONOMERS

Glass ionomers consist of aqueous polymeric acids such as polyacrylic acid, plus basic glass powders. One problem with this type of material is that it leaches out fluoride, as the manufactures believe that fluoride is useful! Use of fluoride- releasing, restorative materials significantly inhibits decay between tooth surfaces next to filled teeth, according to findings from a study published in the June 1999 issue of the Journal of the American Dental Association. This means that if you want a filling without fluoride, you need to ask your dentist. It is also difficult from a dental point of view, as these materials are very useful in deep cavities for reducing post-operative pain.

---

[70] Vimy et al, http://www.bioprobe.com

AMALGAM REPLACEMENT

According to the International Academy of Oral Medicine and Toxicology (IAOMT), there is a protocol for mercury/silver filling removal. They recognise mercury toxicity from various sources such as diet, environment and/or amalgam fillings. The priority in amalgam removal is to ensure that further exposure to mercury by the patient, staff and dentist is minimised. They recommend 8 steps to reducing exposure. [71]

Keep the filling cool during removal.

Use high volume evacuation (aspirator/suction).

Provide an alternative air supply (Many surgeons use oxygen from the anaesthetic trolley and a nosepiece).

Immediately dispose of the mercury alloy. As the particles of amalgam are removed they can lodge in the soft tissues and should be washed away immediately. There is discussion as to whether a rubber dam should be used for amalgam replacement. Some evidence exists that mercury vapour builds up behind the rubber dam. I find clinically that some patients cannot tolerate the dam, while others prefer it.

Lavage and change gloves. After the filling has been removed, the dam and gloves should be removed and the area washed for 30 seconds.

Immediately clean the patient. Debris can get onto the skin of the face and lips. This should be removed.

Nutritional support.

Keep the room air pure using ionizers and fans.

---

[71] Safety in the Dental Office. IAOMT protocol,
www.emporium.turnpike.net/Pdha/mercury/iaomat.htm

PRE-AMALGAM REPLACEMENT [72]

This program should be started two weeks prior to first amalgam replacement.

Glutathione: One 50 milligram capsule upon waking or 30 minutes before breakfast and 1 hour before supper or prior to going to bed.

Cysteine: One 500 milligram capsule twice a day on the same schedule indicated for glutathione. However, it should be noted that in some individuals starting with more than one capsule of cysteine a day, a contra-indication may be indigestion. Therefore, start out taking only one capsule upon waking for three or four days. If no indigestion problems are experienced then add the second capsule. The importance of adding cysteine to your detoxification program is explained succinctly by Braverman and Pfeifer in the following statement:

"Glutathione contains cysteine, glycine and glutamic acid, but of these, only cysteine ever manufactures glutathione whenever extra cysteine is available. Blood glutathione levels change in direct proportion to the amount of cysteine in the diet." [73]

Vitamin C: One 500 milligram tablet with each meal. Clinical experience has shown that in some individuals Vitamin C can affect the way in which they respond to dental anaesthesia. In some patients, the dentist is unable to anesthetize the work area at all. Therefore, as a general guideline, Vitamin C should not be taken for the 12 hours prior to the scheduled dental appointment.

Zinc: One 15 – 30 milligram tablet after supper.

Selenium: One 50 microgram tablet (or liquid equivalent of sodium selenite) taken with each meal.

Vitamin B1: One 50 milligram tablet with each meal.

---

[72] Levenson, J, British Society for Amalgam-Free Dentistry, Brompton Health, 225 Old Brompton Road, London, SW5 0EA
[73] Levenson, J, ibid.

B Complex: Should provide at least 15 – 25 milligrams of each of the various B vitamins. Take the number of tablets indicated to provide the desired amounts.

Magnesium: One tablet per day, providing 100 milligrams of elemental magnesium. Maybe taken at bedtime.

Acidophilus capsules, powder or liquid: Take before going to bed and on waking. May also be taken between meals.

DECISIONS, DECISIONS!
The decision to have amalgams replaced should not be taken lightly. While it may appear the obvious line of treatment to take, there are practical considerations. Many teeth have already been heavily filled. The removal of the amalgam may result in a great deal of work being required with no guarantee of success. Extensive filling removal, leaves very little tooth to fill. These broken-down teeth need root fillings, crowns or extraction. Having the tooth crowned brings with it the difficulty in choice of material. If you are attempting to make your mouth metal-free, then this will include the crowns. Many crowns used today have a metal base with porcelain coating. Out of preference, all porcelain, non-metal crowns are advisable. Composite crowns may be an option but there are questions about long-term durability.

Discussion with a dentist sympathetic to your condition should allow you to decide on the appropriate treatment plan for you.

BLACK TO WHITE
One advantage of the white fillings over amalgam is minimal cavity preparation. I am often asked by patients just why their teeth fracture. One reason that I give is simply that of cavity preparation. When I was a student and amalgam was the only route, we were taught Black's classical cavity designs. Because amalgam is retained mechanically, the cutting has to be made with undercuts to hold the filling in. There are two problems associated with this. The first is the unnecessary removal of sound tooth tissue in order that the filling is retained. The second is that the undercuts can weaken the cusps. In time these cusps fracture. More drilling, more filling, more tooth loss!

LESS TOOTH REMOVAL

The advent of white (composite) fillings and minimal tooth preparation has revolutionized dentistry. The problem is that we've been told that white fillings aren't as strong as amalgams and that there is more chance of further decay.

There is no doubt that white filling placement is more difficult and takes more time. Post-operative pain occasionally occurs in teeth that had no previous history of pain. This of course leads to patient dissatisfaction. These fillings may not last as long as amalgam, but it is hoped that they are not as toxic! Trading longevity of filling for health of the body doesn't seem too great a trade-off. However, materials are improving, as is placement technique.

DUPED DENTISTS

It may be worth considering that the unsuspecting dental profession has been duped too! We learned how to relieve pain and suffering using materials we believed did no harm to the patient. After all, this was our brief. The idea was to solve a problem, not create another one. Yet here we are, looking at materials that would appear far from safe, with the dental profession generally supportive of them. We learned it in school, it must be right! How we cling to our teaching.

DENTISTS INHALE MERCURY VAPOUR, YUMMY!

In research on dental aspirators (suction), it was found that after 20 minutes of continuous aspirator operation, dentists were breathing in mercury vapour concentrations of ten times the current occupational exposure limit.[74] A build-up of amalgam contamination within the internal corrugated tubing of the aspirator was found to be the main source of the mercury emissions, followed by particulate amalgam trapped in the vacuum motor. As the vacuum motor heated up with run time, mercury

---

[74] Stonehouse, C and Newman, A.P, "Mercury Vapour Release From a Dental Aspirator", 26th May 2001. Summarised by B Eley, Professor, Dept of Periodontology, GKT Dental Institute, London

vapour emissions increased. The research points out that the risks from mercury vapour are greater for dentists than for the patients.

The main risks of mercury exposure from amalgam usage occur from mercury spillage, amalgam particle contamination of the surgery, exposure during amalgam placement, removal or cutting, release from mechanical triturators and release from dental aspirators.

WHO'S A MUG THEN?

So, who's the mug? Who's been duped into working with a material that is a known neurotoxin, poison and regular bad guy? Yet dentists throughout the world put their lives at risk and, it would appear, unknowingly. Academics have had their common-sense wings clipped at dental school, convinced by the learned professional bodies, such as the ADA and the BDA, that everything is fine. We use the best materials and, since mercury has been used for 150 years, it must be okay! Hmmmm.

This is not the opinion of leading mercury scientist, Dr Haley, who refutes the ADA in Congressional testimony. He states that mercury is a well-known, potent neurotoxicant, and common sense would lead to the conclusion that severe neurotoxins would exacerbate all neurological disorders, including Parkinson's, ALS, MS, autism and Alzheimer's (AD). Several research papers in refereed, high quality journals and scientific publications have clearly demonstrated that mercury inhibits the same enzymes in normal brain tissues as are found in AD brain samples.[75]

LET COMMON SENSE PREVAIL

In June 2001, a coalition of public interest groups sued the American Dental Association and the California Dental Association, claiming that these organisations had misled the public over the dangers of mercury in tooth fillings.[76] The lawsuits, filed in the Los Angeles Superior Court, are the latest salvo in a growing battle over mercury fillings. The lawsuits allege violations of California's

---

[75] Dr Hayley Refutes ADA in Congressional Testimony
http://www.mercola.com/2001/jun/2/mercury-fillingsdoubts.htm
[76] http://www.mercola.com/2001/jun/27/mercury-fillings.htm

'business and professions code' and charge that the ADA and the CDA have issued rules preventing dentists from discussing the dangers of mercury with patients.

SHALL WE CALL IT 'SICK DENTIST SYNDROME'?

So here we have it. Not only are the patients at risk but also the dentists. On his web page, Dr Rob Gammal poses the question: Are dentists healthy? [77] According to the Journal of Canadian Dentistry, we are a pretty unfit bunch, plagued by the very materials we use to put your teeth right. [78]

Dentists have twice the rate of glioblastoma (brain tumour) than the rest of the population and twice the divorce and suicide rate. IQ psychomotor and psycho-emotional tests score less than average, compared with the rest of the population. Of all the dentists who currently have a long-term disability, 20% are away from their practice because of mental or nervous problems.

Perhaps if we group these 'illnesses' together as one syndrome, then it will get noticed. How does, 'Sick Dentist Syndrome' sound? The dental careers literature might read:

"Smart, fit, dexterous young people wanted, to follow a career that could result in losing your mind. Only those with a short term memory need apply!"

STAFF PROTECTION IN THE US

In the US, OSHA recognises the need for staff protection. It requires that employees be given written informed consent before the use of any toxic chemicals, of which mercury is one. Elemental mercury vapour is one of the most toxic forms of mercury and should not be inhaled. Women of childbearing age shouldn't be exposed to more than 10% of MAC. [79]

Women who are pregnant should be exposed to no mercury. If you use mercury or remove it in any form, the

---

[77] Gammal, Dr Robert, *Guide to Safer Dentistry*, www.gammaldent.htm
[78] *Journal of Canadian Dentistry*, May 1994; Vol. 60, No. 5.
[79] OSHA Job Health Series: "Mercury", (2234)8/1975

National Institute of Occupational Safety and Health (NIOSH) has recommended that your employees be medically monitored on an annual basis. The acceptable level of mercury in the surgery according to OSHA is 50mg/cubic meter. One out of 7 Californian dental offices tested over this level. 100% of the vacuum cleaner exhaust tested over 100mg/cubic meter. According to this report, levels as high as 4000mg/cubic meter have been measured 18 inches from the drill when used dry on an amalgam filling.[80] It is hazardous to the dentist and the patient. If you are looking for a non-hazardous, non-toxic environment in which to work, dentistry doesn't look good, does it?

WHO ARE WE TRYING TO KID?

It appears however that mercury toxicity only occurs in certain parts of the world and not others. A UK Department of Health report begs to differ. The Department of Health Committee on Chemicals in Food, Consumer Products and the Environment on the Toxicity of Dental Amalgam were asked to advise the Medical Devices Agency on the toxicity of dental amalgam.

The Committee consider that their former conclusions are unchanged with regard to the rare occurrence of hypersensitivity and the lack of risk of systemic toxicity.

INADEQUATE DATA

The Committee concluded that: *"There is no evidence that the placement or removal of amalgam fillings during pregnancy was harmful. However, the Committee noted that the toxicological and epidemiological data was inadequate to assess fully the likelihood of harm occurring in such circumstances, and concurred with the view that it may be prudent to avoid, where clinically reasonable, the placement or removal of amalgam fillings during pregnancy."*[81]

---

[80] OSHA MAC is Threshold Limit Value of 100microrgrams/cubic meter or 100ppm. This is the 'never to be exceeded' limit.

[81] Statement by The Committee on Toxicity of Chemicals in Food, Consumer Products and the Environment on the Toxicity of Dental Amalgam. UK Dept of Health, 1998 http://www.doh.gov.uk/hef/amalgam.htm

AMAZING!

It's a miracle! As you cross the Atlantic, West to East, mercury becomes inert, and by the time you put down at Heathrow, this wonderful green island of Britain has purified amalgam fillings to the point where they do no harm. Safe in the Old Dart, your teeth and life are once more secure on the hallowed turf of this fine land. As the flight heads out over Europe, the toxic effects recur somewhere over the channel and by the time the French coast is in view, this inert substance is once again a neurotoxin, frowned upon in Germany and Austria and actually banned in Sweden. If you're not confused, you ought to be! Then again, maybe 'the powers that be' have had too many amalgam fillings and have suffered a lowering of their IQ.

Dr Robert Gammal, past President and now Secretary of the Australian Society of Oral Medicine and Toxicology, has this to say about amalgam:

"When I started to read the scientific literature, I would ask how it is that the universities are still teaching us to use this material and not warn us of the dangers. Surely they would not try intentionally to mislead us? It is inconceivable that this may be possible. After all, we have put great faith in our professors and deans who surely should know the difference between safety and danger and have the moral obligation to tell the truth. Sorry folks, but it is time to change the paradigm and realise that all research and tenured university positions must be paid for. It is time to realise that even the professors have things to lose by not towing the official party doctrine." [82]

VACCINATION

Does this sound too far fetched? Mercury is a known neurotoxin. Why would our professors advocate it? Where else would we use such a substance except in thermometers and sphygmomanometers? You only need to read *World Without AIDS* to understand just how wrong we can get it. Day and Ransom highlight the use of vaccines considered to be necessary to prevent sickness that are themselves potentially fatal. Hepatitis B vaccine

---

[82] Gammal, Robert, ibid.

contains mercury (thimerosal) as well as aluminium and formaldehyde.

Thimerosal is a mercury-containing preservative that has been used as an additive in biologics and vaccines since the 1930's, because it prevents bacterial and fungal contamination, particularly in multi-dose containers. On 20th October 1999, the Advisory Committee on Immunization Practices reviewed information about thimerosal in vaccines:

"Given the widely acknowledged value of reducing exposure to mercury, vaccine manufacturers, FDA and other PHS agencies are collaborating to reduce thimerosal content of vaccines or to replace them with formulations that do not contain thimerosal as a preservative as soon as possible without causing unnecessary disruption to the vaccination system."[83]

Earlier in the same year 27th August 1999, the American Medical Association stated that:

"With the recent concern over the presence of thimerosal in the hepatitis B vaccines, thimerosal-free hepatitis B vaccine is now available.... Unfortunately, because of the current limited supplies of the single-antigen, thimerosal-free hepatitis B vaccine, and in order to ensure prevention of perinatal and early childhood hepatitis B, priority will be given to newborn infants for this thimerosal-free vaccine." [84]

VACCINE-INJURED CHILDREN

In Washington DC, The National Vaccine Information Centre, the oldest and largest organisation in the United States representing vaccine consumers and parents of vaccine-injured children, were calling for the elimination of the mercury content in hepatitis vaccine. [85]

---

[83] Recommendations regarding the use of vaccines that contain thimerosal www.cdc/epo/mmwr/preview/mmwrhtml/mm4843a4.htm
[84] American Medical Association, "Thimerosal–free hepatitis B vaccine available now" http://www.ama-assn.org/ama/pub/article/1809-2071.html
[85] NVIC Press release on thimerosal in vaccines and newborn Hep. B recommendation. http://www.909shot.com/thimersolpr.htm

The point of mentioning thimerosal is that this known neurotoxin is now recognised by the AMA and other official American bodies as being harmful to life. *Yet we in the dental profession still persist in using it in the mouth.*

WHY RISK IT?

Why take the risk? Why use a harmful material when there are now suitable substitutes? The medical fraternity is at least doing something about mercury. Surely the dental profession must follow suit. Why not move on instead of holding on to the sacred cow? Countries such as Sweden have banned the use of mercury, including amalgams, as there are substitutes available. Why not the BDA and the ADA?

MULTIPLE STRESSORS

Stressor upon stressor added to the system, the body battling to cope with the onslaught of drugs, pills, potions and medicaments all supposedly used to improve the quality of life. As we move on now to look at treatments and preventatives, we will continue to witness the dangers of man's intervention.

The Root of the Problem

"A founder member of the Association of Root Canal Specialists discovers evidence that root canals damage your health." [86]

Root canal therapy is the cleaning of the canal that runs up the middle of the tooth. In incisors, there is only one canal, while in molars there are usually three or four. These canals are opened up and files are used mechanically to clean and shape the canal. Once cleaned, the canals are irrigated with various medicaments, dried with paper points and a temporary sedative dressing is inserted.

Once the infection is under control, the tooth is reopened, recleaned and the canal is filled, using a sealant. The actual technique varies from practitioner to practitioner, but essentially the theory is the same. Get rid of the infected material and fill up the cleaned canal with a suitable filling material.

This has been fine for most dentists and many, many people have enjoyed more years from a tooth that could otherwise have been lost. But not all root fillings work. A percentage end up in the dentist's bucket. In root canal practice, we have a technique that is forever being refined and patients who still have their own teeth. So what's the worry over root canal treatment?

Dr George Meinig writes about research covering thousands of experiments, indicating that root canal therapy could weaken your immune system, and could lead to serious illness. Should you have root canal therapy in your mouth? Most dentists rely on information they receive from the ADA, but what if the ADA acts like a trade guild, whose main interest is in its members, and not you? What if they have been suppressing vital information? What if the information they put out is one-sided? *"It seems to us that their actions regarding the controversy over mercury in fillings is a strong indication of this possibility."* states Jerome Mittelman DDS, in his foreword to Dr Meinig's book.

---

[86] Mittelman, J S, DDS, FAPM, past President, International Academy of Nutrition and Preventive Medicine. Meinig, G, *Root Canal Cover–up*, ibid.

THE ESTABLISHMENT
"The position of the American Dental Association and American Association of Endodontists is that root canal fillings are safe." [87]

The British Dental Association states that root fillings cannot save every tooth. First-time root fillings are usually successful and can last many years. If a root filling fails and there is infection again, the root can sometimes be re-filled. But why, if the root filling has been carried out and has enjoyed a measure of success, does it get re-infected? What happens in the body for this to occur?

When decay causes a tooth to become infected and abscessed, dentists are usually quite successful in cleaning out the root canal and disinfecting it. [88] Once this has occurred, the bone loss caused by the infection is replaced. In spite of the seeming success of root canal therapy, Dr Weston Price discovered that bacteria penetrating the dentine tubules had not been killed by the treatment.

ROOT CANAL SEASON
I returned to England from Australia in the fall of 1996. It was interesting to note that the onset of the winter heralded the start of the root canal season. This is the time of year that the endodontically-minded dentist welcomes - open season on pulp removal! This is marked by an increase in the need for root fillings, and the failure of existing root canal work. Why does this happen? Whilst I do not at this moment have research to back up this observation, it appears that, as the health of the community is challenged by the harsh winter months, the immune system can no longer cope with the root-filled teeth and infection or re-infection occurs. This could point to residual infection in the tooth that flares up when the body is compromised.

---

[87] American Association of Endodontists,
http: 12.107.100.106/rootcanalmyths.html
[88] Meinig, George E, *Root Canal Cover-Up*, ibid.

BACTERIA REMAIN IN TEETH

While there is heated debate about whether or not we should root-fill teeth, the one thing believed by both sides is that bacteria remain in the teeth even after they have been root-filled.

Dr Price contends that the 30% of people who enjoyed good health years after root canals had excellent immune systems. He went on to say:

"Nevertheless, when these same healthy people suffered a severe accident, flu, redundancy or stress, which overtaxed their immune system, they could develop a degenerative disease problem because their defences were overwhelmed." [89]

THERE'S A HOLE IN MY TOOTH, DEAR LISA...

It's so big that the decay is through to the nerve. With what shall I fill it?

Decay or bacterial infection insults the nervous and vascular tissue in the root canal, causing inflammation of the pulp. The swelling that occurs causes a constriction at the apex of the root where the vascular bundle enters the tooth, and death of the nerve ensues. Sometimes this is a painless experience with the patient unaware that anything has happened. More often it is accompanied by severe pain.

At first, there is a fleeting pain in the tooth, followed by sharp shooting pains up into the tooth, which explode into the brain. Often the patient will arrive at the surgery clutching a bottle of cold water in an attempt to reduce the pain - sipping occasionally and holding it against the cheek until the liquid warms up. The process is repeated *ad infinitum*. This is "drive-you-crazy" pain. This means extraction of the tooth or a root canal filling. The other condition that requires root canal therapy is usually trauma-induced, where the tooth has been fractured and the nerve is exposed.

---

[89] Meinig, G, ibid.

DEVASTATING THE BODY

As dentists, we have all accepted root canal treatment as standard and are taught how to carry them out. Once a tooth has been damaged to this extent, root canal treatment is the only way, short of tooth removal. Many people enjoy their own teeth for much longer due to the diligence of their dentist. Trained in the mechanics of root canal therapy, we have been unaware of potentially far-reaching health risks associated with root canals.

While the root canal may have been carried out to perfection, the X-ray spot on, and the result excellent, toothache gone, trauma over and the tooth restored to its former glory, there is a hitch. It may be that the very thing we are doing in order to preserve one tooth is actually having a devastating affect on the rest of the body.

ROOT CANAL OR SYSTEMIC HEALTH?
THIS IS THE QUESTION

In his book *Root Canal Cover-Up*, George Meinig DDS, FACD explores the work of Dr Weston Price on:

"Root canals and their possible effects on the systemic system."[90]

Working under the auspices of the ADA, Dr Price and his sixty researchers based their ideas on the focal infection theory. This theory stated that a person could have an infection in one place and the bacteria involved could be transferred, by way of the bloodstream, to another gland or tissue and therein start a new infection.

Dr Frank Billings found that ninety-five percent of focal infections started in the teeth and tonsils.[91] I saw a patient recently who has suffered chronic fatigue syndrome and ankylosing spondylitis. His ear, nose and throat surgeon recommended and then undertook a tonsillectomy in an attempt to cure these problems. The surgeon believed that this patient's systemic problems could be attributed to focal infection. Price's team

---

[90] Meinig, George, ibid.
[91] Meinig, George, ibid.

published 25 papers dealing with the effects of dead or endodontically treated teeth producing other diseases and disorders in remote areas of the body.

BEDRIDDEN CRIPPLE

Dr Price had a patient suffering arthritis who had a root filling. Although the X-ray looked good, he decided to extract the tooth and then embed it under the skin of a rabbit. Two days later the rabbit developed the same arthritis as the patient, It died of infection ten days later. The patient, who was a bedridden cripple, recovered to the extent that:

"She could walk around her house without even a cane and was able to do beautiful, fancy needlework."[92]

Price stated that if the patient had kidney trouble, then the rabbit would develop kidney trouble. If eye failure was noted in the patient, it would also be noted in the rabbit. And it was to be the same with other organs.

When George Meinig read this, he felt that he needed to tell the world of the work of Weston Price. Meinig, an endodontist himself and founding member of the American Association of Endodontists, laid his whole professional career on the line to go against the tide of opinion and publish his work. He says in his book:

"Millions of people are ill, suffering from degenerative diseases for which the medical profession is at a loss regarding cause and treatment; the degenerative disease problem continues to bankrupt our people and country."[93]

He felt that the public should be alerted to the possible effects of root canals and the work of Weston Price.

---

[92] Price, Weston A, ibid.
[93] Meinig, G, ibid.

DISPROVED CLAIMS

The American Association of Endodontists - the same body that George Meinig helped to found, [94] disagrees with the work of Price. It states that subsequent microbiological and epidemiological studies disprove the claims that extraction of endodontically treated teeth could restore the systemically ill person to good health.

They then go on to say that, despite decades of research contradicting the findings of Price: *"One author is attempting to keep the theory alive and recommends extraction of endodontically treated teeth."* Assuming that this author was Dr Meinig, he actually states in his book:

"From all that has been presented, I imagine that most readers will conclude Price was in favour of extracting all root canal-filled teeth and would never consider treating one. You will be pleased to know that this is not what he recommended. Price states, "Don't jump to the conclusion that all root-filled teeth should be extracted.... I do believe that there is a limit of safety for all such teeth for each and every patient." [95]

STRESS CONNECTION

This position is similar to that of Selye, who stated:

"Stress is the non-specific reaction of the body to any demand placed upon it and that this stress is cumulative." [96]

For those with an excellent immune system, root fillings are not necessarily a problem, but those with a low physiological adaptive range may be in more danger.

NATURAL TEETH ARE BEST, EVEN WHEN DEAD!

The American Association of Endodontists suggests that, as good as replacement teeth are, there's nothing as good as a natural

---

[94] American Association of Endodontists
http://107.100.106/ss00ecfe.html
[95] Meinig, G, ibid.
[96] Selye, H, *Stress Without Distress*, ibid.

73

tooth. Endodontic treatment has been proven time and time again to be a safe and effective way of preserving the patient's natural dentition for many years. In this report, they then take the spotlight off root canals and shine it on periodontal disease and its apparent association with infective endocarditis, cardiovascular disease, stroke, diabetes, respiratory disease and adverse pregnancy outcomes. We will be looking at periodontal disease later.

PATIENT-BASED SOLUTION

What approach can we use? I remember treating a lady in Australia who suffered bizarre symptoms following a fall down the stairs. She was referred to me for amalgam replacement. I had almost completed the course of treatment when she came in to see me. Her two front teeth were fractured, the nerves exposed and she was in great pain. I had read Dr Meinig's book and as she had so many other things wrong, I suggested that staying congruent with the treatment so far, it might be better to extract the teeth. Horror replaced her usual smile and with no hesitation she stated:

"I'd rather die than lose my front teeth. This is absolutely not an option!"

OK, SO IT'S VANITY. SO WHAT?

I thought this reaction was a tad over the top, but she'd got her point across. I sat and listened. She could cope with the theory of amalgam replacements, but when it came to the crunch, the loss of her front teeth was more than she could cope with. We saved the teeth with root fillings and she was happy. So while in theory, extraction might sound okay, the needs, desires and wishes of the patient should be met if this is possible.

Since then, I have listened to and seen many people who should lose their front teeth, purely because they are rotten. They just haven't been able to come to terms with the idea of such a drastic solution to their problem and would rather save them at almost any cost than have them removed. As dentists, we need to respect this and look for a biological alternative.

BIOLOGICAL DENTISTRY

Biological dentistry looks at the need for bio-compatibility of filling materials. Conventional dental procedures offer a technique which does not take into account this bio-compatability and the potential for injury to surrounding tissues, due to the caustic nature of the medicaments used and the high percentage of residual bacterial contamination. Dr Boyd Haley of the University of Kentucky says that:

"75% of root canal teeth have a residual bacterial infection remaining in the root. These lingering infections produce toxic wastes that enter the blood stream and can affect any part of the body." [97]

Sound familiar? Isn't this what Dr Price was saying?

IT'S ALKALINE

If the tooth is to be saved, then perhaps biological dentistry has the answer using biocompatible materials. Biocalex, a root canal sealant, has been used in France for over 20 years. It consists of calcium oxide and zinc oxide. It is bactericidal and bio-compatible, with an alkaline pH similar to surrounding tissues. It addresses the poor seal obtained by conventional therapy and eliminates anaerobic organisms. Expansion of the material, as it is converted to calcium hydroxide, seals dental apertures, including necrotic dentinal tubules. It is also more effective than paramonochlorophenol at destroying anaerobic bacteria. [98]

LIVING TISSUES ARE ALKALINE

This is in contrast to Gutta Percha which contains cadmium. This is used as the conventional root canal filling. It is toxic and gives a fairly poor mechanical seal. This is set into place with Eugenol cement, which is acidic, whereas the living tissues are alkaline. The root canal is irrigated with hydrogen peroxide which is caustic to the tissues. It is interesting to note that even with root canals, there is a need to keep the area alkaline.

---

[97] *Biological Dentistry, Health and Happiness*: A newsletter for better living, Volume 4, No. 2. http://www.icnr.com/BiologicRootCanal.html

[98] Biocalex. Bio-Probe Inc. http://bioprobe.com/biocalex/index.asp

CHOICES, CHOICES

To treat or not to treat? That is the question. If saving the tooth is a priority, then the biological approach would appear to have solved the dilemma of both parties. The importance of nutritional supplementation needs to be stressed at this point. If you, the patient, want this treatment to succeed, then it would be a good idea to build up the body with great nutrition.

If you are contemplating root canal therapy, please read the nutrition section at the end of this book to ensure that you are in the best condition to receive this treatment.

Camel Breath and Bleeding Gums

They have numerous TV advertisements for body odour. I think they ought to have some for mouth odour. Maybe I'm just super critical but after over twenty years in dentistry, I still don't like bad breath. So often, I observe people hiding behind a hand, too embarrassed to laugh, too self-conscious, almost defeated by the fear that their breath smells and that their teeth look dreadful. Yet many do nothing about it. We know the stigma of bad breath and a yucky mouth. But it is also a health risk and a potential cause of systemic disease.

MEMORIES

As a child, I remember the overbearing maths teacher from school, who would lean in a little too close and then breathe his fetid odour over me, whilst explaining the mysteries of algebra and geometry. Then there was the round, cuddly, sanguine female friend of the family who would love me, hug me, squeeze me and plant such malodorous kisses on my unsuspecting cheek - kisses that I could smell for a week.

NOT SO SWEET

I remember an elderly alcoholic lady who attended surgery for tooth removal and the fitting of full dentures. I had to bribe her into the surgery with the promise of a Scotch after the ordeal. Of course with a mouth like hers, there was a lot of blood and general foulness of odour. The job done, dentures inserted into the mouth, she dismounted and planted a great big juicy, slobbery, bloody kiss on my face. Oh, the joy of dentistry. How could I ever complain? Anyone want to be a dentist?

SAY IT, DON'T SPRAY IT!

Perhaps for you, it was the wonderful salesman looking for his last deal to close the day and make his target. No water for a whole day, just coffee, stale aftershave and gum to hide his bad breath. Would you really want to buy anything from him? All lovely people I'm sure, but all people that you don't want within arm's length. Say it, don't spray it: give the news not the weather: hear it, not wear it: conversation, not precipitation, etc., etc. These are the people who, if they couldn't knock you down with a look, would certainly deck you with a single outward breath!

SYSTEMIC AILMENTS
Poor oral hygiene, bleeding gums, bone loss and bad breath are indicators of potential systemic ailments. The endodontic fraternity have apparently denied any link between root-filled teeth and systemic disease (as stated by the American Endodontic Association).[99] They do recognise however that there is a growing body of epidemiological evidence that seems to support the premise that non-endodontic oral infections, specifically periodontal disease, appear to be associated with diseases such as infective endocarditis, cardiovascular disease, stroke, diabetes mellitus, respiratory disease and adverse pregnancy outcomes.

In July 1998 the American Academy of Periodontology launched an effort to educate the public about new findings which support that which dental professionals had long suspected:

"Infection in the mouth can play havoc elsewhere in the body. Periodontists know that periodontal disease is a bacterial infection, and all infection is cause for concern." [100]

GUM CONSTRUCTION
The periodontium is made up of gum, root surface, connective tissue attachments and bone. The healthy gum looks pink, firm and stippled in texture. It appears to adhere to the enamel surface of the tooth and the mouth looks healthy. In gum disease, the gingiva changes in colour, becomes puffy and bleeds easily with brushing or light pressure. Often when you brush your teeth, as you spit out the toothpaste, it is discoloured with blood from the inflamed gums. This is gingivitis, which occurs when the bacteria, which exist normally in the mouth, proliferate, increasing in mass and thickness to form a plaque. J D Lindhe, MD, Ph.D defines plaque as:

---

[99] American Association of Endodontists, "Oral Disease and Systemic Health", http://www.mercola.com/12.107.100.106/ss00ecfe.html
[100] American Academy of Periodontology http:www.perio.org/consumer/mbc.top2.htm

"A bacterial aggregation on the teeth. This causes cellular injury, with subsequent swelling, redness and heat."[101]

INFECTION FIGHTERS

Gingivitis precedes periodontitis. The periodontium is made up of gum (gingiva), root surface (cementum), connective tissue attachments and bone. The tooth sits in a matrix of tissue that allows it to move when load is applied to it. This prevents pain and fracture on biting, as there is a little "give" with pressure.

It is this supporting tissue that breaks down in periodontitis. The plaque hardens when left in place, to form calculus (tartar). This cannot be removed with brushing and requires a dentist or hygienist to remove it with scaling. The trick is to prevent it forming in the first place.

DOWN IN THE MOUTH

It is known that certain medical conditions render patients more sensitive to this inflammatory process, including diabetes and Down's Syndrome. Gingivitis may also flare up a few days before menstruation, when progesterone levels are high. Progesterone tends to dilates blood vessels, causing inflammation, and blocks the repair of the collagen or connective tissue that supports the teeth. Pregnancy gingivitis is also quite common.

FOCAL INFECTION

One of the most important revelations of Dr. Price's research concerned how bacteria in teeth metastasise and, as they migrate throughout the system, go on to infect the heart, kidneys, joints, nervous system, brain and eyes.[102] They can also endanger a pregnant woman and may infect any organ, gland or body tissue. This theory of focal infection was not popular at the time and is still looked at with scepticism. Price showed that endodontically treated teeth caused infection elsewhere in the body. The endodontists tend to disagree and turn the infection over to the periodontists.

---

[101] Lindhe, J D *Textbook of Clinical Periodontology*, Munksgaard, 1984
[102] Meinig, G. ibid.

PASSING THE BUCK

Here we have two specialities of dentistry treating bacterial infection. The endodontists say there is no link between root-filled teeth and systemic disease, but agree with the periodontists that bacteria from periodontal disease may be linked to systemic disease. Jan Lindhe, a renowned periodontist, states that involvement of the periodontal tissue is frequently a result of death of the pulp of the tooth. In the non-vital pulp, micro-organisms find conditions that favour their growth.

The bacteria will release enzymes, metabolites, antigens, etc., which will emerge into the periodontium through canals and foramina that regularly connect the pulp chamber with the periodontal ligament. Once in the periodontium, an inflammatory reaction takes place, destroying the periodontal ligament and resorbing adjacent bone.

HEALTH DANGERS

It would appear from this that both endodontic and periodontal lesions would be dangerous for the health of the individual. This would concur with the position of Dr Weston Price that teeth and gums do affect the systems of the body.

Once the full weight of this concept is realised, then the need for good oral hygiene becomes obvious. Continuous monitoring of the periodontal status of susceptible people must be paramount in the practice of dentistry.

MASSIVE STROKE

A few years ago my father-in-law suffered a massive stroke with occlusion of his right carotid artery. After the controlled panic of packing my wife off to Austria to be with him, I sought the help of nutrition biochemist Dr Serjit Verk. This was the one man I knew I could trust to give me the best information needed to help. We used oral chelation, the antioxidant pycnogenols, a liquid ionised trace mineral and vitamin solution and several other nutritional approaches.

LUCKY TO BE ALIVE

The doctors warned my father-in-law that he would be lucky to live. The stroke had completely paralysed his right side and affected his speech and memory - difficult for a man who can speak at least five languages and who runs his own business. Today, he is very much alive - walking, talking and playing golf!

DENTAL PREVENTATIVE REGIME

Research showed me that there was also a link between periodontal infection and systemic disease. In this case, specifically stroke. I had seen my father-in-law's dental X-rays and I knew that the condition of his mouth was not good with advanced bone loss, periapical infections (infection at the root tip) and gum disease. Amongst the other products that we added to his regime were non-toxic toothpaste and a specially formulated mouthwash. What he needed was good oral/dental care products with no harmful ingredients. These would really help to get the condition of the mouth under control and reduce the risk of opportunistic infection aggravating his present situation. It also made sense to me to put him on the best protection program available.

NUTRITION CONNECTION

Could it be that there is a nutritional link here? We look to oral hygiene as the way of cleaning up the act and preventing premature tooth loss. But as we will see later, in the chapter on nutrition, perhaps the link is not just one of oral cleanliness, but also one of malnutrition. Scurvy manifestations in the mouth are described by French Mariner Jacques Cartier thus:

"Their mouths became stinking, their gums so rotten, that all the flesh did fall off, even the roots of the teeth which did almost fall out."[103]

How often has your dentist talked to you about scurvy? Never, I am sure. But what of nutrition? Are we treating the problem locally without any attempt to treat the obvious systemic disorder? Could it be that gum disease can be reversed, not only by good oral hygiene but also by good nutritional supplementation?

---

[103] Day, Phillip, *Health Wars*, ibid.

POSSIBLE HEALING PROCESS

Could it be that calculus build-up is a healing process, the calcified material being deposited in an attempt to wall up the leaking gums and prevent further tissue breakdown? So far I haven't found any research on this, but it is an interesting thought, especially in light of the knowledge that plaque formation in the arteries (atherosclerosis) is the answer to tissue fragility and the possibility of blood leaking through damaged arterial walls because of the patient's nutritional deficiencies.[104]

STROKE AND GUM DISEASE

In Toronto on 21st April 1999, at the American Academy of Neurology (AAN) annual meeting, it was suggested that periodontal disease may increase the risk of stroke.[105] People with periodontal disease are likely to have thickened carotid arteries, which can lead to a stroke. Fifty-two people who had never had a stroke were given an ultrasound test to determine the thickness of their carotid arteries. The result showed that the people with the most periodontal disease had the most thickening of the carotid arteries. This was enough for me to make sure that my father-in-law increased his levels of oral cleanliness!

Since the doctor/nutrition combination had such a beneficial effect, I don't want him facing this ordeal again, especially if one of the causative factors is dental. It wouldn't go down too well at home, and anyway I like him and want him around for as long as possible, as with all my patients!

It is interesting to note gum disease being linked to a thickening of the carotid artery. Could it be that both are a manifestations of nutritional deficiency?

---

[104] Day, Phillip, *Health Wars*, ibid.
[105] American Academy of Neurologists, "Periodontal Disease May Increase the Risk of Stroke", 51st Annual meeting, 21st April 1999, Toronto, Canada http://www.pslgroup.com/dg/f896a.htm

CUT DOWN ON DENTAL CHECK-UPS
IT SAVES MONEY!

Only this week, we have been given to understand that the routine six monthly check-up is a thing of the past in Britain. According to the Daily Telegraph, check-ups cost the British National Health Service £108 million in the year 2000 and many believe the money could be better spent. As Aubrey Sheiham, Professor of Dental Health at the University of London, says, *"There is no evidence that 90% of adults need to go to the dentist every six months. The majority could go every two to three years."* He says that they are dentally healthier due to fluoride toothpaste. I'm not so sure fluoride is the factor (please see the chapter on fluoride). He believes that costs could be cut by up to £200 million if adults changed from twice a year to once a year. [106]

MOUTH CANCER:
THE CASE FOR REGULAR CHECKUPS

This might be so if the only criteria for a check-up were to examine teeth. In practice, it is not uncommon to see a patient who had a scale only a few weeks ago and then return with yet more calculus to remove. It doesn't take much to persuade the average person to go less often to the dentist. Most would rather not go at all.

The fact is that people need to be monitored for both periodontal health and oral lesions. The latter may be benign, such as Lichen Planus, which presents as white lacy striations on the insides of the cheeks. Lichen Planus is of apparently unknown origin. Occasionally it becomes erosive and is then very painful. It can often be seen next to amalgam fillings. I had a patient in Australia who suffered from erosive Lichen Planus. She did really well after amalgam removal, and the change of all her personal care products to safe alternatives, including her shampoo!

As a money-saving exercise, the government may see it as good policy to reduce dental examinations. However if the American Academy of Periodontists is to be believed, then acting on the dubious privilege of having less check-ups and thereby reducing the

---

[106] "Change in Policy", *Probe Dental Magazine*, April, 2001

incessant pounding on government coffers may leave people at risk of developing gum disease, periodontal disease and systemic disease.

COSTS CUT THROUGH EDUCATION
Cutting back can only come after enough time and education have shown that periodontal disease has been stemmed. As for fluoride toothpaste, the majority on the market not only contain fluoride but also sodium lauryl sulphate.[107] SLS is a well-known skin irritant which breaks down protein. This suggests that fluoride may help the teeth, which, according to some research, is highly doubtful. The SLS in the toothpaste may in fact harm the gums.

Bacterial re-colonisation can occur as quickly as three months after a thorough scale, so cutting back on these check-ups isn't necessarily such a good idea - except as a cost-cutting exercise for government. In clinical practice, three months is often optimistic. I have seen calculus build up over a two-week period, even in patients who think that they are brushing well. What do we do for these people? Do we leave them for a couple of years, or shall we get on with the job in hand?

A survey reported In the annual report by the UK's NHS Dental Estimates Board, London, HMSO (1991/2) of over 4,000 adults, showed 75% of 33–44 year olds had periodontal disease, with some irreversible loss of tooth supporting tissues. 13% had severe forms of periodontal disease. Are these people at risk?

BE RATIONAL
With heart disease still the number one killer and cancer a close second, maintenance of a healthy mouth becomes of paramount importance. It will take a while to educate the public into this new way of thinking about solid nutrition and the mouth and general health connection. Once the realisation comes that tooth brushing, flossing and the use of a mouthwash is more than a social necessity (it is part of the general prevention program), then hopefully more widespread acceptance for a rational treatment plan will materialise.

---

[107] Antczak, Stephen & Gina, *Cosmetics Unmasked*, Thorsons, 2001

VOLATILE SULPHUR COMPOUNDS(VSC'S)

Most people are concerned about halitosis or bad breath. Volatile sulphur compounds (VSC), mainly hydrogen sulphide, methyl mercaptan and dimethyl sulphide, break down the resistant barrier of the periodontium, causing bad breath. As the severity of the periodontal breakdown increases, so too do the volatile sulphur compounds. By eliminating these compounds, there is the potential to control periodontitis and eliminate bad breath. This also increases the validity of the prevention program.

Professor Perry Ratcliff at the University of California believes that the active ingredient, stabilised chlorine dioxide, neutralises the VSC's, which may help in preventing and treating active periodontitis. [108]

Check-ups are important, as is the advice of the dentist or hygienist, but they are not with you all the time. Nothing can replace a good toothbrush, toothpaste, floss and a mouthwash, unless the toothpaste and mouthwash contain harmful ingredients. According to leading toxicologist Dr Samuel Epstein:

"The amount of irritation caused by toothpaste is minimal but can include sore mouth and gums, wearing away of tooth enamel, sore tongue, and sloughing of mucous membrane." [109]

It is claimed that toothpastes containing both sodium lauryl sulphate and Triclosan continue working for up to twelve hours. The American College of Toxicology reports:

"Both sodium and ammonium lauryl sulphate appear to be safe in formulations designed to be discontinuous, brief use followed by thorough rinsing from the surface of the skin. In products with prolonged contact with the skin, concentrations should not exceed 1%." [110]

---

[108] Ratcliff, P, Research targets a Social Taboo, *Dentistry* 19th October 2000

[109] Steinman, D & Samuel S Epstein, *The Safe Shopper's Bible*, Macmillans, 1995

[110] Chae, Linda, "You Have a Right to Know"
http://lindachae.com/Truth_about_SLS.htm

WHY USE CANCER-CAUSING CHEMICALS?

As Linda Chae points out, twelve hours is not exactly 'discontinuous, brief use'.[111] Triclosan is a chlorophenol - a class of chemicals suspected of causing cancer in humans. Externally, it can cause skin irritation. Internally, it can lead to cold sweats, circulatory collapse, convulsions, coma and even death. Why would you want this working for twelve hours in your body when there are safer alternatives?

MOUTH CANCER

A 1991 survey of people with mouth, tongue, or throat cancers suggests that the use of a high alcohol-content mouthwash contributes to increased risk of tumours. Most of the individuals had used a mouthwash daily for twenty or more years. It is so sad that we use products for years in the belief that we are doing the best, only to find that years later this was never the case. Once again, it highlights the danger of presuming that products used for years are safe. We only need to look at aspirin or Valium to know that we can sometimes get it wrong. Aspirin was used as the panacea for all ills. And while it appears to have done a great job, it can be lethal. We were also taught that Valium was safe and non-addictive. We now know that this is just not the case.

So what can we use to reduce the systemic risk of periodontal disease while at the same time having at least some assurance that we are not harming ourselves in the process? With toxins in our filling materials, and dental care products with harmful ingredients, it is extremely important to pick the right products to keep the mouth healthy, the breath fresh and free from potential skin irritation and carcinogens.

---

[111] Chae, Linda, ibid.

How Much Fluoride Is Enough?

"Water, water, everywhere and not a drop to drink."

If water fluoridation becomes mandatory, will the above be seen as a prophecy come true?

FLUORIDE'S DUBIOUS BENEFITS

"What's with fluoride?" I hear you cry, especially you outraged dentists who believe that any word spoken out against this *saviour* of teeth is tantamount to blasphemy! What's wrong with it? We've been sold the idea that fluoride saves teeth, and, according to the misquoted York report, that it is effective and safe.[112] The same press releases assure us over other supposedly beneficial drugs like Tamoxifen, which is used to combat breast cancer, but is now also reportedly the cause of endometrial cancer.[113] Perhaps we need to look beyond the localised effects of dubious dental benefit and consider the potential destruction caused in the rest of the body by the ingestion of fluoride.

DANGER IN THE BATHROOM

According to Dr Ted Spence, fluoride does the following:

Inactivates 62 enzymes
Increases the ageing process
Increases the incidence of cancer and tumour growth
Disrupts the immune system
Causes genetic damage
Interrupts DNA repair-enzyme activity
Increases arthritis and is a systemic poison. [114]

---

[112] York Review, British Fluoridation Society, www.derweb.co.uk/bfs/york

[113] Tamoxifen is an oestrogen receptor antagonist and, at a daily dose of 20mg, is the hormonal treatment of choice for breast cancer in postmenopausal women. Caution is recommended as an increased incidence of endometrial changes including cancer, has been reported in association with Tamoxifen. *Dental Practitioners' Formulary.* 1998-2000

[114] Spence, E, "The Fluoride Controversy" www.mercola.com/1999/feb/21/fluoride_controversy.htm

All of this can be yours just to save your teeth!

According to Kurttio, fluoride increases the risk of hip fracture.[115] Kurttio and colleagues studied over 144,000 elderly, rural Finnish people admitted to hospitals with their first hip fracture, who had lived at the same address from 1967 to 1980. They found that women aged 50-64 years old exposed to natural fluoride levels greater than 1.5mg/litre had significantly more hip fractures than similar women least exposed to fluoride at 0.1 mg/litre. This disagrees with the Lancet study showing no fluoridation/hip fracture link. Kurttio however said that the Lancet study was flawed since it was not gender-specific.

On the matter of fluoride causing hypothyroidism, Andreas Schuld, head of Parents of Fluoride-Poisoned Children (PFPC), adds:

"The recent discovery of hundreds of papers dealing with the use of fluorides in effective anti-thyroid medication poses many questions demanding answers. The enamel defects observed in hypothyroidism are identical to dental fluorosis. Endemic fluorosis areas have been shown to be the same as those affected with iodine deficiency, considered to be the world's single most important and preventable cause of mental retardation, affecting 740 million people a year, according to the WHO."[116]

FLUORIDE - AN EMOTIONAL GIANT
Maybe we should take off the emotional blinkers. Forget those heady student days when fluoride was *'the thing'*, and take a good look at just what is happening with fluoride today. After all, as dentists you needn't worry. There are enough alternative sources of fluoride in our diet and environment without needing it in our toothpaste and water systems - that is, if you still believe that one part per million is the safe fluoride-ingestion level!

---

[115] "Fluoride Does Increase the Risk of Hip Fracture", *American Journal of Epidemiology* Oct. 1999 http://www.pslgroup.com/dg/16e7fe.htm
[116] www.bruha.com/fluoride/index.html

As students, we were taught that one part per million of fluoride (optimal dose of 1mg of fluoride per day) added to the water was the optimum for good dental health. This was ideal to reduce the level of dental decay and build good strong caries-resistant teeth. Once ten parts per million were reached, there was evidence of fluorosis, characterised by mottling of the enamel, disfigurement with white opacities or brown marks on the teeth. So, if one part per million is optimum, it begs the question as to why the majority of toothpastes contain in excess of 15 parts per million. The great British cup of tea contains 4.57mg per litre, diet coke 1.12mg/l and the average apple 1mg of fluoride.[117]

FLUORIDE BAN IN AUSTRIA

The world's largest study on dental caries observed 400,000 students. It revealed that decay increased 27% with a 1ppm-fluoride increase in the drinking water.[118] In Graz, Austria, dental caries in children increased whilst fluoride tablets were being dispensed. Begun in 1956, decay decreased after they stopped it in 1973. In 1998, the results of a 50-year fluoridation experiment involving Kingston, New York (un-fluoridated) and Newburgh, New York (fluoridated) were published. In summary:

"There was no significant difference in rates of dental decay in children in the two cities, but children in the fluoridated city showed significantly higher rates of dental fluorosis than those in the un-fluoridated city."[119]

TRENDY TRENDLEY

How much fluoride do we need and who spread the rumour in the first place?

In 1939, Dr H Trendley Dean was working for the US Public Health Service. He examined water from 345 communities in Texas. Dean determined that high concentrations of fluoride in the water in these areas corresponded to a high incidence of mottled

---

[117] Schuld, Andreas, "Fluoride in Food", *PFPC*
http://www.bruha.com/fluoride/html/f-_in_food.html
[118] Teotia, S P S, Teotia, M, "Dental caries: A Disorder of High Fluoride and Low Calcium Dietary Interaction", *Fluoride*, 59-66, 1994
[119] Ziegelbacker, Rudolf, "Fluoridation in Europe", *Fluoride* 31 (3), 1998

teeth. He also claimed that there was a low incidence of dental cavities in communities where the water contained 1ppm of fluoride. The 10% who showed mild fluorosis with whitening of the enamel were described as having "beautiful white teeth."

INVALID DATA
Dean's report resulted in fluoridation being implemented at 1ppm. When other scientists tried to verify Dean's results, they disagreed with his findings. He had engaged in the selective use of data, using findings from 21 cities that supported his case, while 272 locations were disregarded. Never let the truth stand in the way of a good story, they say! When taken to court over his findings and put under oath, Dean admitted that his data were invalid. In 1957 he had to admit at AMA hearings that even water containing 0.1ppm (0.1mg/l) could cause dental fluorosis.

This represents good news and bad news. The good news is that fluoride may possibly, but then on the other hand it might not, make your teeth stronger. The bad news is that while we attempt to go for strength, the teeth will look dreadful and you'll end up with tooth reduction and the placement of porcelain veneers in an attempt to cover up your ugly teeth!

It's '...just a cosmetic problem', according to the final report of the British Government-sponsored review into the benefits and adverse effects of water fluoridation, published in October 2000.[120] As stated earlier, even this report was misquoted, according to Professor Sheldon, chairman of the advisory group.[121]

THE YORK REPORT
Sheldon's letter, dated 10th December 2000, reads as follows:

"In my capacity of chair of the Advisory Group for the systematic review on the effects of water fluoridation recently conducted by the NHS Centre for Reviews and Dissemination, I

---

[120] *The Advisory Group for the Systematic Review on the Effects of Water Fluoridation*, NHS Centre for Reviews and Dissemination, University of York UK, Oct 2000.
[121] www.npwa.freeserve.co.uk/sheldon letter.html

am concerned that the results of this review have been widely misrepresented. The review was exceptional in this field, in that it was conducted by an independent group to the highest international scientific standards and a summary has been published in the British Medical Journal.

It is particularly worrying that statements which mislead the public about the review's findings have been made in press releases and briefings by the British Dental Association, the National Alliance for Equity in Dental Health and the British Fluoridation Society. I should like to correct some of these errors.

1. Whilst there is evidence that water fluoridation is effective at reducing caries, the quality of the studies was generally moderate and the size of the estimated benefit, only of the order of 15%, is far from massive.

2. <u>The review found water fluoridation to be significantly associated with high levels of dental fluorosis</u>, which was not characterised as "just a cosmetic issue." [emphasis added]

(According to the British Fluoridation Society's version of the same report, it was stated that the review recognises dental fluorosis as a cosmetic issue, not a health problem, and acknowledged that it occurs in non-fluoridated areas as well as fluoridated areas.)[122]

3. <u>The review did not show water fluoridation to be safe</u>. The quality of the research was too poor to establish with confidence whether or not there are potentially important adverse effects in addition to the high levels of fluorosis. The report recommended that more research was needed. [emphasis added]

(The British Fluoridation Society's reading of the report: *The review was set up to establish whether fluoridation is still effective, and whether it is still safe, and the report is unequivocal: water fluoridation is EFFECTIVE and SAFE.*)

---

[122] York Review: "Questions and Answers", www.derweb.co.uk/bfs/york

4. There was little evidence to show that water fluoridation has reduced social inequalities in dental health.

(Again the BFS states: *the review confirms that water fluoridation reduces inequalities in dental health. It narrows the gap between young children and their more affluent peers.*)

6. Probably because of the rigour with which this review was conducted, these findings are more cautious and less conclusive than in most previous reviews.

7. The review team was surprised that, in spite of the large number of studies carried out over several decades, there is a dearth of reliable evidence with which to inform policy. Until high quality studies are undertaken providing more definitive evidence, there will continue to be legitimate scientific controversy over the likely effects and costs of water fluoridation.

Professor Trevor Sheldon, MSc, DSc, Fmed Sci.[123]

POLITICAL SHENANIGANS
This has all caused a bit of consternation. Here we have the chairman clarifying the report. Yet the pro-fluoridation lobbyists are still claiming the victory to be theirs. The BFS see the results slightly differently from the chairman! On their questions and answers web page, the BFS question 14 reads:

Q. Can the Government press ahead with fluoridation in the light of the findings of the review?

A. The findings of the review are unequivocal; water fluoridation is effective and safe. On the basis of this review, the Government should now demonstrate that it is serious about reducing health inequalities and improving the health of children, and press ahead with the White Paper pledge to: "introduce a legal obligation on water companies to fluoridate where there is strong local support for doing so".

---

[123] Sheldon T, Dept. of Health Studies, Innovative Centre, York Science Park, University Road, York, www.npwa.freeserve.co.uk/sheldon_letter.html

Now, this doesn't exactly agree with Professor Sheldon! How can this be?

NEW ZEALANDER AGAINST FLUORIDE
Perhaps the explanation given by New Zealand dentist John Colquhoun, who was an ardent advocate of fluoride before he changed his mind, will help us to understand. He realised that he and his colleagues were doing exactly what history shows mistaken professionals do when confronted by disconcerting new evidence: *"They bend over backwards to explain away new evidence and keep their own reputations and theories intact!"* [124]

INDIA
In October 1998, Dr A K Susheela, the Director of Fluorosis and Rural Development Foundation, New Delhi, India, presented scientific evidence on; *"The adverse effects of fluoride on human tissues, due to fluoride contamination of drinking water, fluoridated dental products and fluoride therapy."* She pointed out that fluoride is known to cause a variety of health problems, such as dental fluorosis, skeletal fluorosis and non-skeletal manifestations. In India, an estimated 62 million people, including 6 million children, are afflicted with endemic fluorosis. [125]

INDIAN GOVERNMENT
MOVE AGAINST FLUORIDE
This is such a problem in India that, far from adding fluoride to their water, former Indian Prime Minister Rajiv Gandhi set up a program to remove fluoride and other pollutants from the water supply. This is in contrast to the UK, USA, Australia, Canada, New Zealand, Ireland and other parts of the world, where governments continue to add fluoride to the public water supply, in defiance of the overwhelming body of evidence.

---

[124] Colquhoun J, "Why I changed my mind about water fluoridation." *Perspectives in Biology and Medicine*, Autumn 1997
http://www.fluoridation.com/colquhoun.htm
[125] Susheela, A K, "Scientific evidence on adverse effects of fluoride", Fluorosis Research and Rural Development Foundation, New Delhi, India

CANADA

A recent report from the Canadian government questions the value of water fluoridation. On 23rd April 2001, Dr David Locker, a University of Toronto dentistry professor, reports: *"No Canadian studies provide evidence that water fluoridation is effective in reducing tooth decay in contemporary child populations."*[126] After 30 years of fluoridation, decay levels should have levelled off. They haven't! We already know that Dr Trendley Dean was wrong, and in the opinion of Paul Beeber, fluoridation is a big mistake:

"We believe that calcium and other well known bone and tooth building minerals in the water and soils were responsible for lower decay rates, not the fluoride!"[127]

HANKY PANKY

The battle rages. The pro-fluoride machine is well under way with claims that water fluoridation reduces tooth decay, and that the advent of fluoride toothpaste has reduced dental caries. Fluoride is heralded as the saviour of our teeth and mass fluoridation a must. Yet, it would appear, that there might just be some hanky panky going on. If you don't read Prof. Sheldon's letter and only read the pro-fluoridation reports, then you could be forgiven for believing that everything is okay with fluoride. But what about the disastrous effects of sucrose and other refined foods in the diet? Do these get a look-in? Not at all. The political lobby for the sugar industry is proving very able in keeping serious adverse data out of the media.

What about our toothpaste?

DEATH BY TOOTHPASTE!

In 1994, Dr Peter Rock of Birmingham University warned that even a pea-sized quantity of fluoride toothpaste might be too toxic for young children.[128] The year before, a scientist at the Poison Information Centre in Vienna published figures showing that there

---

[126] Canadian Government report questions the value of fluoride. Contact: Paul Connett, Ph.D, Professor of Chemistry, St Lawrence University, Canton, NY, USA

[127] Beeber, Paul, President of New York State Coalition Opposed to Water Fluoridation, www.orgsites/ny/nyscof

[128] Gotzsche, Anne-Lise, "The Poison Smile", UK *Guardian*, 19th October 1995

were 450 cases of fluoride poisoning in children in Austria every year and one death. In Britain, these figures would transfer to 3,000 cases and seven deaths.

In November 1996 the Colgate Palmolive Company in the United Kingdom made a 'goodwill' payment of £1,000, after an independent specialist diagnosed a young boy as suffering from severe dental fluorosis.[129] The belief was that this condition resulted from the use of his toothpaste. The company is marketing a product, ratified by the dental profession, and doing what the profession expects it to do. The fact that the American Dental Association has expressed concern about a dramatic increase in dental fluorosis hasn't stopped the pro-fluoride movement.

Toothpaste companies are simply keeping up with demand in the market place. Yet now there are companies who are manufacturing safe toothpaste and other personal care alternatives with the potentially harmful ingredients removed to encourage the public to move towards non-toxic alternatives in their lives. I praise the efforts of these organisations and encourage them to get their messages out to the public far and wide.

WHAT IS 'FLUORIDE'?
If you did chemistry at school you may remember fluorine as that pale yellow, pungent toxic gas that would make your eyes water. Fluoride compounds are so toxic, they are listed among the top 20 of 275 substances that pose the most significant threat to human health, in the list compiled by the US Agency for Toxic Substances and Disease Registry. (ATSDR). In Australia, the National Pollutant Inventory ranked fluorides as 27 and 28 out of 208. Ranking was given based on health and environmental hazard identification and human and environmental exposure to the substance.

Fluoride compounds are cumulative, systemic toxins. It is for this reason that US law requires the Surgeon General to set a

---

[129] Colgate Palmolive sued for fluoride toothpaste injury. www.nofluoride.com

maximum contaminant level for public water supplies. This is aimed at avoiding crippling skeletal fluorosis.[130]

ACCUMULATION WITH NO DOSE CONTROL

Remember, Selye said that stress is cumulative. To reduce stress, the stressors or cumulative toxins need to be reduced. If this is so, then why do we need controlled fluoride in our water supplies? We already have uncontrolled fluoride in our toothpaste, mouthwashes, foods and pesticides. And we also have contaminants that enter our food chain via our crop treatments or indirectly through rain water entering our water supplies and then being sprayed onto our gardens to help vegetable growth. These represent more accumulation of toxins, leading to disease.

We need to consider the total amount of fluoride ingested from all sources. According to Dr Paul Connett, Professor of Chemistry:

"If 1ppm. was considered to be optimum for drinking water in 1945, it cannot be considered optimum for today, because there are far more sources of fluoride available and unavoidable (processed food, fruit juices, toothpaste, etc). To claim that 1ppm is optimum for today is to underline the unscientific nature of the pro-fluoride lobby." [131]

At the end of this letter, Dr. Connett stated that these are his own views and should not be read as being endorsed by either his department or university.

EXPOSURE TO FLUORIDE

Exposure to fluoride comes not just from toothpaste, fluoride tablets, topical fluoride application and slow fluoride emission from filling materials placed by your dentist. It also comes from airborne fluorides and from many diverse manufacturing processes. These include pesticide applications, phosphate fertiliser production, aluminium smelting, uranium enrichment facilities, coal burning

---

[130] "What is Fluoride?" www.bruha.com/fluoride/index.html

[131] Connett, Paul, Professor of Chemistry, St Lawrence University. Canton, New York 13617. Letter to Ray Jones, Chairman of Operations and Environment Committee, City of Calgary, 8th August, 1997
www.fluoridation.com/calgary1.htm

and nuclear power plants, incinerators, glass etching, petroleum and vehicle emissions, insecticide sprays, some aerosols and even teflon pans! Even medication used for depression, such as Prozac, (one of the range of serotonin uptake inhibitors) is fluorine-based. Fluoride is everywhere. Fluoride compounds, either organic or inorganic, have been shown to exert anti-thyroid effects.

The first Parents for Fluoride Poisoned Children (PFPC) newsletter states:

"We have learned that the major iodine-deficient areas of the world are identical to endemic fluorosis areas. We have learned that in some endemic fluorosis areas, hypothyroidism, as a result of iodine deficiency, affects over 50% of all children. We have learned that one child dies every minute due to complications associated with this fluorine-induced iodine deficiency, and that this is a problem affecting a third of the population, perhaps more." [132]

CANCER RISK

In his discussion on why he changed his mind about fluoride, John Colquhoun cites bone cancer as another reason for not using fluoride. It has been found that osteosarcoma, a rare bone cancer, has dramatically increased in young human males. This increase has been found in boys aged 9-19 in fluoridated areas of America, but not in non-fluoridated areas. [133]

WARNING! WARNING!

Epidemiological studies of cancer, especially the bone cancer (osteosarcoma) in the US, have shown a positive link to fluoride. This is supported by animal studies. There are also links with congenital anomalies, Down's Syndrome, foetal and brain damage causing low IQ, due to fluoride passage across the placenta. This and other extracts were taken from *'Some Scientists and*

---

[132] PFPC newsletter, No 1, 1st November, 1999, www.orgsites.com/ny/nyscof

[133] Hoover, R N, Devesa, S, Cantor, K, Fraumeni, J, "Time trends for Bone and Joint Cancers and Osteosarcomas", US Public Health Service, 1991

Professionals Opposed to Fluoridation'.[134] Dr Paul Connett states that:

"While the authors of the study on osteosarcoma do not claim that their work is definitive at this point, it is a huge warning signal which would be imprudent to ignore." [135]

Dr Dean Burk, co-founder of the US National Cancer Institute, is none too keen on fluoride, stating: *"Fluoride causes more human cancer death and causes it faster than any other chemical."* [136] These are warning signals that cannot be ignored! We have known since 1944 that fluoride was unsafe. The Journal of the American Medical Association published an editorial stating that the use of drinking water containing as little as 1.2 to 3 ppm of fluoride will cause developmental disturbances in bones such as osteosclerosis, spondylosis and osteoporosis, as well as goitre.[137]

DEBATED IN THE HOUSE

In the UK House of Lords, they are still unsure of the weight of this world-wide research. They appear to be debating whether we should fluoridate British water or not. There is as much confusion in the Upper House as there is within the British Fluoridation Society. In a written answer, dated 17th January, 2001, Lord Hunt of Kings Heath stated:

"The York review showed that fluoridation does reduce dental decay and found no evidence of serious adverse effects on oral health. But there was lack of high quality research. We have therefore asked the Medical Research Council how it might be possible to strengthen the evidence currently available."

---

[134] Foulkes, Richard, www.fluoridation.com/calgary1.htm
[135] www.fluoridation.com/calgary1.htm
[136] D'Raye, Tonita, "The Facts About Fluoride", PO Box 21075, Keizer, OR 93707 USA.
[137] *Journal of the American Medical Association*, "Health-damaging Effects of Fluoride", Oct 1944. A list of some thirty clinical trials demonstrating the adverse effects of Fluoride compounds on bone is kept on file at Credence and CTM.

IF YOU DON'T LOOK, YOU WON'T FIND

The York Review considered only fluoride exposure from water fluoridation. It did not examine the total fluoride exposure of populations from all sources, as advised by WHO. The narrow criteria of the review resulted in the exclusion of all animal studies, all biochemical studies and all mathematical and statistical models, effectively eliminating from the review a vast body of scientific evidence attesting to the harmfulness of fluoride via exposure from water and a wide variety of other sources.[138] This is not the way to inspire confidence among the electorate.

WHAT IS MORE IMPORTANT: TEETH OR GENERAL HEALTH?

It is interesting that the report only mentions oral health, but not systemic health. Of particular concern is the exclusion of a substantial body of peer-reviewed scientific evidence on *"The serious effects of fluoride on the thyroid gland."*[139] Are we attempting to improve dental health at the expense of general health? It would appear so, just by virtue of the fact that there is still consideration being given to fluoridating our water supplies.

We want healthy teeth but at what price? We also want the right to smoke if we like but more and more evidence suggests a link between smoking and cancer. Even passive smoking is a danger. If there is any question about the safety of fluoride, it must be up to the individual to make a personal choice. We must have the right to choose and not allow the government to enforce mass medication through water fluoridation.

ENVIRONMENTAL POLLUTANTS

We have already established that fluorides are dangerous to public health. The fluorides used in the drinking water are toxic and non-biodegradable, are environmental pollutants and are officially classified as contaminants by the US Environmental Protection Agency. The two main culprits are hexa(hydro)fluorosilicic acid and sodium silicofluoride. These chemicals are industrial waste by-products from the manufacture

---

[138] www.npwa.freeserve.co.uk/sheldon_letter.htm
[139] www.npwa.freeserve.co.uk/sheldon_letter.html

of phosphate fertilisers and the aluminium industry, removed from the recovery filters of their pollution scrubbers.

BETWEEN A ROCK AND A HARD PLACE

This puts us somewhere between a rock and a hard place. Nowhere to go and with little room for manoeuvre. Even with this information available, many governments and the dental profession are still bent on compulsory water fluoridation. Even to the scientific mind, this is unbelievable. And for those blessed with a modicum of common sense, it is crazy. If you want fluoride, if you believe in fluoride, if fluoride makes you tick, then you can get it so easily without contaminating our water supply. For those who still want fluoride, it is readily available in toothpaste, mouthwash, fluoride tablets, floss and, of course, the great British cup of tea. You don't have to miss out.

IS THERE A SOLUTION?

According to Dr Hardy Limeback, head of Preventive Dentistry, University of Toronto and President of the Canadian Association of Dental Research, he had told his colleagues and students that he had unintentionally misled them.

"For the past 15 years, I had refused to study the toxicology information that is readily available to anyone. Poisoning our children was the furthest thing from my mind." [140]

Among the findings that changed his mind, was the realisation that in fluoridated areas, hip bones had double the fluoride content as compared with non-fluoridated areas, causing skeletal fluorosis and weakening of the bone.

OPEN AND HONEST

What do we do instead? If there are even just suspicions that fluoride is harmful, then this must be enough for it to be given a full and open examination.

---

[140] Limeback, Hardy, www.lindachae.com/fluoridenews.htm

THERE ARE SAFE ALTERNATIVES

1. **Education and nutrition**. In Birmingham, England, tooth decay was related to socio-economic status. The answer is not fluoride but good nutrition. If sucrose causes tooth decay, then it makes sense to reduce it, not add fluoride.

2. **Non-fluoride toothpaste**. For the last eight years, I have been using a non-fluoride toothpaste and have recommended it to everyone who I meet. It contains no harmful ingredients and no fluoride. Its active ingredient is anthium dioxide.

3. **Mouthwash.** Again, there are great and safe alternatives which need to be promoted by dentists and the public alike.

4. **Toothbrushing and flossing**. Many people brush, but few floss their teeth. With advancing years, brushing alone is not enough. As the bone levels sink around the teeth and you become 'long in the tooth', there may well be a need to floss.

BE GROSS, SNIFF THE FLOSS

Floss removes the grot from between the teeth. If you don't think you need it, try the sniff test. Run the floss between the teeth, remove it and smell it. If it's as sweet as a rose you're doing well; if it is odorous, you know that you need to floss. Many people do not like the idea of floss, but get over it and get on with it. If I can do it, you can do it!

In summarising this chapter, I would like to turn again to Dr Susheela, who states:

"Fluoride enters the bloodstream within minutes after tooth brushing with fluoride toothpaste." [141]

We have seen from the research that fluoride negatively affects health. In those who use or ingest fluoride, it has been observed that muscles and bone tissue undergo degenerative changes. This in turn leads to tooth loss. Fluoride may well be one of the factors

---

[141] "Serum and Urine Fluoride Levels in Toothpaste Users", *Journal of the Indian Dental Association*, Vol. 59, June-Sept, 1987

responsible for us becoming edentulous. What started off as a good idea has in all probability been a major cause of tooth loss and degenerative disease. Now that we have safe choices, there is no further need to expose ourselves to these harmful toxins.

Brush and Swill
(An overview of toothpastes and mouthwashes)

Warning: *Keep out of reach of children under six years of age. If you accidentally swallow more than is used for brushing, seek professional help or contact a poison control centre immediately.*[142]

You might be forgiven for believing that you have just read the label on a household poison or some cleaning material that you brush onto your floors or work surfaces; products that you keep locked in a cupboard away from the children. However, this is the warning on an American toothpaste packet.

POISON CENTRE
A known poison, left in the open for all to see and encouraged to use – and be sure to use at least twice a day. You can put it in your mouth, brush with it, swill it around, write on the mirror with it, but dare swallow this frothy solution and you are instructed to contact the local poison centre! What comfort, what joy to know that you have to supervise your child, while you knowingly allow him/her to use and perhaps ingest a potent toxin. Even if you could keep the toothpaste out of harm's way, you still have to educate the man of the house. Who isn't beyond leaving the top off the tube, squeezed from the middle, dribbling down the side of the basin and lying in a messy pool just south of the plughole? To be fair, most cases of fluoride toxicity have followed accidental ingestion of insecticides or rodenticides (rat poison), but as a tale of caution, if there are safe alternatives, why entertain the risk?

THE HISTORY OF TOOTHPASTE
Powdered ashes of hooves of oxen, myrrh, powdered eggshell and pumice.

Nothing like a bit of ox hoof to keep your teeth clean (I thought the expression was dog's breath). This was the Egyptian answer to

---

[142] Crest toothpaste carton warning, Proctor and Gamble, Cincinnati, OH 45202, USA

oral hygiene a few thousand years before Christ. It did get better though. They used a toothpowder containing hart's horn, burnt shell of snails, oysters and gypsum. They went on to use dried animal parts, honey and powdered flintstone. Toothpowders and pastes were developed in Britain in the late eighteenth century. The contents of these products were often harmful and abrasive to the teeth. They used china, brick dust and cuttlefish.

In 1873, Colgate introduced an aromatic toothpaste and later, a dental cream. Soap was then added as an emulsifying agent. This was not effective and tasted dreadful and was replaced by sodium lauryl sulphate. Basically, toothpastes have moved on from ingredients that sound as if they can kill you, to chemicals that can indeed kill you.

PLAYING HOOKY
A trick used by the Austrian school children on the day of an exam was to swallow some toothpaste. Within twenty minutes they would develop a temperature that would enable them to stay at home with good reason. Some would additionally get headaches, nausea and vomiting, but as this only lasted a couple of hours, it was considered worth the inconvenience.

So what are the ingredients in toothpaste that cause the trouble? We have already gone into detail on sodium fluoride, but I think it is worth summarising some of the more salient points with regard to this and other common substances used in personal care products.

SODIUM FLUORIDE
Sodium fluoride is found in most toothpastes in concentrations of up to 1500ppm. Let us remember the research article of Dr Susheela, stating that: *"Fluoride from these toothpastes enters the circulation within minutes."*[143] This is a significant finding, Dr

---

[143] Susheela, A K, "Scientific Evidence On Adverse Effects of Fluoride", presented to Members of Parliament and The Lords, House of Commons, Westminster, London, October 1998

Samuel Epstein stating: *"The use of fluoride in toothpastes is controversial because of suggestive evidence of carcinogenicity."*[144]

In 1993, the U.S. Public Health Service published a lengthy official document called *'Toxicological Profile for Fluorides, Hydrogen Fluoride and Fluorine.'* It included the following:

"Populations that are unusually susceptible to the toxic effects of fluoride (and its compounds) include the elderly, people with deficiencies of calcium, magnesium and Vitamin C and people with cardiovascular and kidney problems. Fluoride is excreted through the kidney, so people with renal insufficiency would have impaired clearance to fluoride. Impaired renal clearance of fluoride has also been found in people with diabetes mellitus and cardiac insufficiency. This decreased clearance of fluoride may indicate that elderly people are most susceptible to fluoride toxicity. Inadequate levels of magnesium may affect the toxic effects of fluoride. As fluoride levels rise in the body calcium levels go down." [145]

DEATH BY TOOTHBRUSHING

Maybe I missed the lecture on who should and who should not use fluoride toothpaste, but I can't remember any mention of the fact that there is a certain section of the population that really ought to be advised against using toothpaste containing fluoride. Imagine being treated for a kidney complaint or just getting on top of your cardiac insufficiency, when you mistakenly swallow a mouthful of fluoride toothpaste. You are defeating the whole exercise with your oral hygiene program. Can you imagine the coroner's report? *"Death by toothbrushing."*

SODIUM LAURYL SULPHATE

Sodium lauryl sulphate is a synthetic detergent derived from coconut oil.[146] It functions as a denaturant, detergent, emulsifier and surfactant. It is used widely in shampoos, cleansing lotions,

[144] Steinman, D & Epstein,. S, *The Safe Shoppers Bible*, ibid.
[145] Jones J, (Campaign Director, National Pure Water Association) *Halifax Evening Courier*, Saturday, 31st October, 1998
[146] Antczak, Stephen and Gina, ibid.

foaming bath oils, toothpastes and liquid soaps, shaving cream, shower gel, facial cleansers, baby wipes, hand and body creams and many other products.

EYE DAMAGE

Sodium lauryl sulphate can cause contact eczema, eye and skin irritation. In studies carried out by Dr Stephen Green, SLS was found to penetrate eye tissue and cause retinal damage for up to five days.[147] What about children with SLS in their shampoo? Further studies suggest that SLS prevents children's eyes from developing properly, possibly by denaturing the protein in the eye and inhibiting correct structural formation. It would appear that this damage is permanent and also suggests that there is retardation of healing in eyes when exposed to SLS. In 1983 it was reported that animals exposed to SLS experienced eye damage, depression, laboured breathing, diarrhoea, severe skin irritation and even death.[148] Prolonged use in bath oils can lead to irritation of the mucous membranes of the genitals, resulting in urinary tract and vaginal infection.

PROTEIN BREAKDOWN

As sodium lauryl sulphate is protein-denaturing, its use can result in epithelial desquamation - the sloughing off or loss of skin.[149] This means that the use of SLS toothpastes in susceptible people may result in loss of the top layer of the mucous membrane inside the mouth with resultant soreness or even ulceration. It may also produce cracking of the dermal and epidermal layer of the skin.[150] It has been my observation in practice that people can react quite badly to their toothpastes. Mouth ulcer sufferers should change to a toothpaste with no harmful ingredients. I also encourage the use of ionised minerals, vitamins and trace elements to help stabilise the body.

---

[147] Green, Stephen, "Detergent Penetration into Young Adult Eyes". Courtesy of *Research to Prevent Blindness*, 1985
[148] *Journal of the American College of Toxicology*, 1983
[149] Fakhry Smith, S, Din, C, Nathoo, S A, Gaffar, A, "Clearance of Sodium Lauryl Sulphate From the Oral Cavity", *Journal of Clinical Periodontology*, 313-317. 24th May 1997
[150] "SLS", *Journal of Investigative Dermatology*, www.lindachae.com

There is also a link between SLS and cancer. While it apparently does not of itself cause cancer, when mixed with other common ingredients, it can become carcinogenic.

WARNINGS UNHEEDED

Dr Stephen Antczak sums up this substance very well in his book *Cosmetics Unmasked*. He says:

"And why was sodium lauryl sulphate the most common cleaning chemical in shampoos, shower gels, foaming bath oils, and everything else that cleans? The bottle on my laboratory shelf carries the following list of warnings:

Avoid inhaling the dust.
Wear suitable protective clothing.
Irritating to eyes, skin and the respiratory system.
Harmful by inhalation or if swallowed.
May cause sensitisation by inhalation.
May cause serious damage to the eyes.
In the event of eye contact, rinse with plenty of water and seek medical advice.

Did I really want this stuff in my toothpaste?" [151]

If commercial toothpastes are so bad, what's the alternative? We still want to brush our teeth, have fresh breath and reduce or prevent tooth decay. Brushing alone is insufficient to remove bacteria from all aspects of the teeth, especially in the contact areas. The use of anti-bacterial agents in the toothpaste would appear to be necessary.

TOOTHPASTES: THE NEW BREED

There is a new breed of toothpaste in the marketplace. Its active ingredient is anthium dioxide, manufactured from chlorine dioxide, sodium carbonate and sodium bicarbonate. *"It is very safe, non toxic and is FDA, EPA, and USDA approved to disinfect, clean up and purify."* says Tom Mower, Research Biochemist and President of Neways International, which has developed Radiance

---

[151] Antczak, Stephen and Gina, *Cosmetics Unmasked*, ibid.

toothpaste and Eliminator mouthwash, both these products using anthium dioxide as the active ingredient. [152]

ANTHIUM DIOXIDE
Volatile sulphur compounds (VSCs) comprise hydrogen sulphide, methyl mercaptan, and dimethyl sulphide. They help to break down the resistant barrier of the periodontium, causing malodour. As the severity of the breakdown increases, so too does the presence of the VSCs. By eliminating these compounds, there is the potential to control periodontitis and eliminate bad breath.[153] Anthium dioxide is very powerful at breaking down sugars and other food films and removing the odours they can cause. It is also a powerful disinfectant for the bacteria in the mouth.

Professor Perry Ratcliff, who has used chlorine dioxide technology to develop Retardex oral rinse, spray and Retardent toothpaste, states:

"Chlorine dioxide has a very high bacterial kill rate and can be used for long term treatment and maintenance of bad breath." [154]

According to Scotmas, which markets anthium dioxide as the complete water treatment, chlorine dioxide is widely regarded as a far superior biocide to chlorine, which cannot be used in the mouth. The properties and advantages of chlorine dioxide over chlorine are as follows:

"Removes bio-film and thoroughly cleans tanks and pipes, removing the threats from bacteria and other infection. It does not produce chlorinated by-products and carcinogens, as a result of disinfections. It is not dependent on pH, and can be used in alkaline systems. It has a broad-spectrum biological kill pattern, including all bacteria, spores, viruses, fungi, cysts and protozoa. It acts against foul-tasting compounds in water systems, such as

---

[152] Mower, Tom, Neways International, Salem, Utah, USA. Written letter dated 13th July 1994
[153] Jaroodi, Jane, *Dentistry*, 19th October 2000
[154] Ratcliff, Perry, University of California, San Francisco

hydrogen sulphides, chlorinated compounds and phenols, oxidising them to tasteless, odourless compounds." [155]

Using this technology allows us to move away from the products with potentially harmful ingredients, and start employing toothpastes that really work.

BAD BREATH

In the healthy mouth, more than 350 species of micro-organisms have been found. Periodontal infections are linked to fewer than 5% of these species, and inflammatory lesions do not erupt in the absence of these bacteria. When there is a change in oral hygiene status or it is abandoned, the aerobic bacteria - the good guys - are replaced by anaerobic bacteria, which are found in periodontal disease. Bad breath is due to the breakdown of proteins by these anaerobic bacteria. Their waste products are sulphur-based. It is those volatile sulphur compounds that smell.

There are also local reasons for bad breath. These include:

Foods: garlic, onions, eggs, cheese, mints, etc.
Drinks: coffee, tea, alcohol, milkshakes, beer, etc.
Medication: many medicaments give bad breath, often due to the drying effect on the oral mucosa.
Sickness: the mouth dries out, the bacteria increase in activity and sulphur deposits appear as a white covering over the tongue.

---

[155] www.Scotmas.com

The Danger of Chronic Dehydration

A dry mouth smells the worst. There are medical conditions that lead to drying of the mouth. However, we most commonly experience it after a night on the town, a great meal, a bottle of red wine, washed down with coffee and brandy, then to bed. Semi-comatose, snoring heavily, mouth open and dry, we awake with a mouth which feels, I am reliably informed, like the bottom of a parrot's cage - a delightful aroma, sure to bring romance into the bedroom first thing in the morning! The alcohol and coffee dry the mouth and, in the absence of oxygen-rich saliva, the anaerobic bacteria proliferate to release the pungent odour.

AGGRESSIVE RADIOTHERAPY

I recently treated a patient with rampant caries. The decay in his teeth had been caused by his dry mouth. This dry mouth (xerostomia) was brought on by aggressive radiotherapy to kill off his cancer. Radiation-induced xerostomia causes degeneration of the salivary glands in proportion to the amount of parotid gland irradiated.[156] With his salivary glands shot to pieces, his only relief was found in the bottle of water that was with him constantly to quench the unpleasant side effects of his therapy. When he was well enough, he would attend treatment and I would fill what I could. The next visit would reveal more decay and more and more, we were fighting a losing battle in his mouth and he, for his life.

He later died of the cancer that had consumed his body. The treatment intended to relieve him of his cancer had left him uncomfortable, distressed and had decimated his quality of life. Treating mouth cancer with the conventional approach carries a 50% death rate. Early diagnosis is the key to any chance of survival.[157]

---

[156] Rose, Louise F & Kaye, Donald, *Internal Medicine for Dentistry*, ibid.
[157] High death rate of oral cancer,
http://www.lineone.net/skynews/uk/story/1999/9/c—1999-9-25-4n4.html

Radiation is not the only cause of a dry mouth. The Californian Dental Hygienists' Association has reported that xerostomia may be caused by:

"... a number of medical conditions which may be temporary (such as anxiety or dehydration associated with diarrhoea) or permanent, as in Sjogren's syndrome, or "unavoidable" damage to the salivary glands during radiotherapy." [158]

INDUCED BY MEDICATION

Sometimes a patient may complain of a dry mouth when saliva production is normal. Although xerostomia is often associated with the elderly, advanced age itself is not the cause of a dry mouth. However, older patients have a greater likelihood of having a medical condition associated with xerostomia or there is an increased probability of them taking medication known to cause a dry mouth as a side-effect. This dry mouth may be an unrecognised contributing factor in periodontal disease and tooth loss in three out of ten adults.[159] The treatment prescribed for this condition is, of course, good oral hygiene with regular visits to the hygienist, the elimination of sugar-free sweets or gum, plus a number of other products on the market that have been developed to resemble saliva and its antimicrobial constituents.

SALIVA IS WATER-BASED

Nowhere in this report is water mentioned. Yet saliva is water-based with inorganic ions and contains several hundred different proteins.[160] A dry mouth is the last outward sign of dehydration. Dr Batmanghelidj's book opens our eyes to the possibilities of the simplest cure for many diseases that hound our society today. During his three years' imprisonment in Iran, he treated and cured over 3,000 ulcer cases with only water – the element we all take for granted - the element that the medical profession has dismissed as unworthy of research!

---

[158] Lewis, Michael A O, "Xerostomia: Not Simply a Dry Mouth", *The Dentist*, April 2001

[159] Xerostomia. Dental Hygienist Supplement, *The Dentist* Vol. 17, No 4, April 2001, George Warman Publications Ltd, www.gwarman.co.uk/dentist

[160] Robinson, Colin, "Saliva", *Dental Digest*, Vol. 1, Issue 1, October 2000

Dr Batmanghelidj says in his book:

"Since my eyes were opened to water as a natural medication, I have developed and applied this technique to the point where it has alleviated and healed hundreds of traditionally incurable sicknesses and chronic pains. I have seen water completely reverse conditions such as asthma, angina, hypertension, migraine headaches, arthritis pain, colitis pain, chronic constipation, heartburn and hiatal hernia, depression, chronic fatigue syndrome, high cholesterol, morning sickness, overweight problems – even heart problems thought to need bypass surgery. All these conditions have responded simply and permanently to water. Ordinary "natural" water. Any water you feel comfortable drinking is fine. Clean [non-polluted] *tap water is as good as any."*[161]

TURN ON THE TAP

From his book we can understand just how overlooked water is, and yet we are 75% water. The new scientific truth and level of thinking about the human body that will empower people to become practitioners of preventive medicine for themselves is as follows: it is the solvent – the water content - that regulates all functions of the body, including the activity of all the solutes (solids) that are dissolved in it. The disturbances in water metabolism of the body produce a variety of signals, indicating a system disturbance in the particular functions associated with the water supply and its rationed regulation. Simply said, if we don't have enough water, then the body rations water on a priority basis and the system goes into dysfunction.

DEHYDRATION

It is now possible to understand the dry mouth, not as some strange phenomenon, but for what it is - a sign of dehydration. When I ask patients how much they drink, mostly they say, *"Plenty!"* This 'plenty' turns out to be several cups of coffee, a cup of tea, maybe a juice with breakfast and a glass of wine or beer in the evening. In this there is no mention of water. For some, the only water they get is the ice melting in the gin and tonic. We have not

---

[161] Batmanghelidj, F, *Your Body's Many Cries For Water*, ibid.

been brought up to appreciate water. Even in school, we were encouraged to drink milk at break time, but water seemed unimportant. It is not difficult to go through a day without drinking one glass, yet Dr Batmanghelidj recommends at least 8-10 eight ounce glasses a day. That's a couple of litres or more *daily*. So if you're feeling sluggish, or your body is on go-slow, or maybe it's toxic and turgid, or maybe you have acute, chronic pains, consider that the body is unable to function in its dehydrated state.

Why is it that the elderly complain of a dry mouth? Sometimes it can be medication-induced. But Dr Batmanghelidj's explanation makes far more sense:

"It is now becoming obvious that, from an early adult age, because of a gradually failing thirst sensation, our body becomes chronically and increasingly dehydrated. With increase in age, there is a gradual and steady loss of sensitivity of the thirst sensation and insufficient water intake will alter the ratio of the amount of water held inside all the cells to the volume of water held outside the cells of the body. The water we drink will keep the cell volume balanced and the salt we take will maintain the volume of water that is held outside the cells and in circulation. As a result of this chronic dehydration, symptoms that equal disease are seen. The problem appears to be that while we are dehydrated, we don't realise it. Our thirst button has been turned off. While our body is crying out for water and the mouth is obviously dry, there is no appreciation of the thirst or the need to satisfy it." [162]

TREAT ONE CONDITION, CAUSE ANOTHER

So where are we getting this water from? Dr Batmanghelidj says that clean tap water is as good as any. So long as our water hasn't been pre-medicated and is pure, this statement holds true. But if we drink fluoridated water while we are hydrating, we are subjecting the body to a chemical attack - a fairly common medical phenomenon, where, in treating one condition, we cause another. It is akin to using diuretics for essential hypertension in a patient whose hypertension is caused by chronic dehydration. Essential hypertension says Dr. Batmanghelidj:

[162] Batmanghelidj, F, ibid.

"...should primarily be treated with an increase in daily water intake. The present way of treating hypertension is wrong to the point of scientific absurdity. The body is trying to retain its water volume, and we say to the design of nature in us: "No, you do not understand – you must take diuretics and get rid of water!"

Many illnesses, which plague millions of people worldwide, spring from a simple unrecognised cause – we don't drink enough water.

COFFEE AND SODA NOT THE ANSWER
Dr Mercola writes that most people fall short of recommendations to drink eight 8-ounce servings a day. Although nearly three quarters of Americans are aware of the recommendations, only 34% actually drink this amount, while 10% said that they do not drink water at all. However, Americans drink an average of nearly six servings a day of caffeinated beverages, such as coffee and soda. These drinks can actually cause the body to lose water, making proper hydration even more difficult to attain. Caffeine, one of the main components of the many different sodas on the market, is a drug. It is addictive because it has a direct action on the brain. It also acts on the kidneys, increasing urine production. Physiologically, it is a dehydrating agent - the more you drink the more you need. This is great for the drink companies, but is a major player in causing an increase in weight.

REAL WATER – THE ANSWER
Dr Mercola states: *"Your exclusive beverage should be water. Bottled spring water is best, but filtered water is acceptable. Try to have a least 8 glasses of water a day. It would be best to have water at room temperature. Ice cold water can be a trauma to the delicate lining of the stomach, unless you are overheated."* [163]

Dr Batmanghelidj states that the body needs an absolute minimum of six to eight 8-ounce glasses of water a day. Alcohol, coffee, tea and caffeine-containing beverages do not count as water.

---

[163] http://www.mercola.com/2000/june/10/watewr.htm

The best times to drink water (clinically observed in peptic ulcer disease) are: one glass 30 minutes before taking food and a similar amount two and a half hours after food. I have found that it's a good idea to watch your water intake. It's really easy to believe that you're taking enough, only to realise at the end of the day that you've fallen short. It is easy to replace coffee or tea at work with a cup or two of water. In the winter, warm to hot water is a pleasant drink once you've got used to it. In one practice, I received really odd looks when the coffee order came round. I had the coffee with no coffee, no milk and no sugar. Hot water only! In my job there is also the practical application. The two breaths most unpleasant for patient and dentist alike are those exhaled by the coffee drinker and the smoker.

BREATHING DIFFICULTIES

When I first arrived in Queensland, I was amazed at the number of children suffering from asthma. It seemed like we had walked into an epidemic. Endless numbers of children were walking around, all sucking on their inhalers. It is probable that I hadn't noticed the asthmatics in England. In the UK, 3.4 million people suffer from asthma, killing at least 2,000 people a year. [164] It is said that asthma is a common disease in which the circular smooth muscles of the branching air tubes of the lungs - the bronchi - are liable to go into spasm (broncho-spasm), so that the bronchi are narrowed and the passage of air impeded. It is often easier to breathe in than out and the lungs become inflated and cannot easily empty. An exhaling wheeze is a regular feature of an asthma attack. The commonest kind is allergic asthma, but asthma can also be induced by infection, emotion, occupational hazards and exertion.

SALT AND WATER

According to Dr Batmanghelidj, asthma is not a disease that needs to be cured. It is a physiological adaptation of the body to dehydration and salt shortage. It will recur whenever insufficient attention is paid to regular water and salt intake. A pinch of salt on the tongue after drinking water fools the brain into thinking a lot of salt has arrived in the body. It is then that the brain begins to relax

---

[164] http://ds.dial.pipex.com/sean/asthma/

the bronchioles. Alcohol and caffeine contribute to severe asthma attacks. People with asthma should slightly increase their salt intake. With so many people suffering this condition worldwide, surely this simple measure cannot be ignored.[165]

EXPAND NARROW DENTAL ARCHES AND OPEN AIRWAY

One of the problems encountered by functional orthodontists is breathing difficulties. Mouth-breathing children with narrow dental arches and a forward head posture suffer particularly in this area. Often these children also complain of asthma. Whilst we in the dental profession have spent our time looking at structural correction of the mouth (in conjunction with physiotherapists, chiropractors and osteopaths who concentrate on skeletal corrections to upright the head on the spine), simple recommendations such as increasing water intake have more often than not been overlooked.

REDUCE VSC WITH WATER

Often the presentation for dry mouth is bad breath. Usually the spouse has complained and the partner has to see if anything can be done. They have used a variety of toothpastes and mouthwashes, but all to no avail. Scaling and polishing the teeth gives some help, as does the use of a non-alcohol mouthwash. The only treatment for the dehydration is water. Once the body is rehydrated and salivary flow re-established, the volatile sulphur compounds (VSCs) produced by the anaerobic bacteria will reduce. We need water, we need it clean and we need it in quantity. However, according to Paul Beeber:

"Dentists are unknowingly endorsing arsenic and lead into our drinking water. Without residents' consent, dentists in little towns, big cities and some states convince trusting legislators to add fluoride into the water supplies, claiming it reduces tooth decay. However, the fluoride treatment chemicals used are

---

[165] BBC online http://www.bbc.co.uk/health/asthma/

contaminated with lead, arsenic and other industrial by-products." [166]

According to the National Sanitation Foundation (NSF), the only three chemicals certified for fluoridation are: hydrofluosilicic acid, sodium fluoride and sodium silicofluoride. *"...The most common contaminant detected in these products is arsenic,"* reports the NSF. *"The other significant contaminant found is lead."*[167]

Beeber adds: *"We understand the considerable expense it takes for communities to remove naturally occurring arsenic from water supplies; but it is unconscionable that water engineers are allowed purposely to add lead and arsenic-contaminated fluoride into water supplies without consumers' knowledge or informed consent, at the urging of mis-informed dentists."* [168]

TOXIC WATER OPPOSED
The US Environment Protection Agency Headquarters Union of Scientists opposes fluoridation. They took their stand based on the scientific literature documenting the increasingly out-of-control exposures to fluoride, the lack of benefit to dental health from ingestion of fluoride, and the hazards to human health from such ingestion. These hazards include acute toxic hazard, impaired kidney function, cancer, reproductive effects, neuro-toxicity, bone pathology and dental fluorosis.

EVEN PRO-FLUORIDE DENTISTS
DOUBT BENEFITS OF FLUORIDATION
The EPA has also found that the tide of opinion is turning against fluoridated drinking water. Statements are now being issued by dentists in the pro-fluoride camp who are warning that topical fluoride (e.g. fluoride in toothpaste) is the only significantly

---

[166] Beeber, Paul, "Dentists Unknowingly Endorse Arsenic and Lead into our Drinking Water. NYS Coalition Opposed to Water Fluoridation", www.orgsites/ny/nyscof
[167] Hirzy, William Ph.D, "Why US EPA'S Union of Scientists Opposes Fluoridation". Copies available from the National Pure Water Association, www.npwa.freeserve.co.uk
[168] Beeber, Paul, ibid.

beneficial way in which fluoride affects dental health. In any event, a person can choose whether to use fluoridated toothpaste or not (although finding non-fluoridated kinds is getting harder and harder), but one cannot avoid fluoride when it is put into the public water supplies.

The water issue is too important to ignore. The body needs good, clean water. The unsuspecting public however is drinking the sorry alternative, believing it will do no harm. How can we encourage our patients and friends to drink more water when it is being tampered with in so disgraceful a manner?

DEHYDRATED DENTAL NURSE

Tanya came to work for me just recently. She had been working in a florist's shop, but had to give up due to asthma and hay fever. She was taking two different antihistamines, one three times a day and the other once a day. She started drinking water on her first day of work at our surgery. Within two weeks, her asthma and hay fever had disappeared. She has since come off her medication and hasn't had any need for her inhaler. The headaches that plagued her have stopped altogether. One could argue that moving out of the florists could have reduced her symptoms, as also the reduction in coffee. However, she continues with the water and enjoys this very effective treatment for her condition. She is now a waterholic, rather than a caffeinholic and she's feeling great!

SIMPLE, CHEAP AND THIRST-QUENCHING

We have a simple, cheap, non-invasive and effective treatment for a dry mouth. Good oral hygiene can be maintained by the use of non-fluoridated toothpaste, mouthwash and water. Once we understand the importance of water and add it to the daily routine of life:

"... billions of dollars could be lopped from the annual health-care budgets in all advanced countries, greatly reducing our dependence on manufactured drugs from the pharmaceutical companies." [169]

---

[169] Batmanghelidj, F, ibid.

A not uncommon complaint amongst my patients, especially the elderly, is one of a dry mouth. They have no known medical condition, nor have they undergone any destructive therapy, but they are aware of dryness, even when the mouth appears moist. In the past, this condition had been a difficult one for me to treat and in the main, I took the easy way out and referred them back to their general medical practitioner. Now I look forward to helping the many people for whom a dry mouth and a dehydrated, scaly, lethargic body are a real problem.

ALCOHOL

It has already been established that alcohol dries the mouth, reducing the oxygen concentration and increasing anaerobic activity. Why then would you use it as a mouthwash? You end up getting the very thing that you are trying to prevent, which is bad breath. The effect of the freshening of the breath with this alcohol-based product is short-lived and replaced by a dry mouth. Some of the leading brands contain alcohol at up to 27% or 54% proof. This is somewhere between a Jack Daniels at 43% and wine at 12.5%. Do you really want your children using this?

DRUNK IN CHARGE OF A TOOTHBRUSH

On 30th October 1997, the Crown Prosecution Service won its High Court appeal against a court decision not to ban a mouthwash addict from driving after he was found to be nearly three times over the drink-drive limit.[170] Mr Jowle pleaded guilty to consuming excess alcohol, but said he had become addicted to Listerine earlier in the year, unaware that it contained alcohol. The magistrate decided not to impose an otherwise mandatory driving disqualification after hearing that Listerine contained 26.9% alcohol by volume, although there was no indication of its presence on the bottle.

MOUTHWASHES ASSOCIATED
WITH CANCER IN WOMEN

In the *Safe Shoppers Bible*, it is suggested that mouthwashes with high alcohol content should not be used:

---

[170] "Mouthwash Driver Facing Ban After Perverse Court Decision Overruled", www.lineone.net/skynews/uk/story/1997/10/c

"A 1991 survey of people with mouth, tongue or throat cancers suggests that the use of high-alcohol mouthwash contributes to increased risk of these tumours. Most of the individuals surveyed had used mouthwash daily for over twenty years. The increased risk was only seen in people who used mouthwashes with 25 percent or higher alcohol content. This study agrees with a report in the 1983 Journal of the National Cancer Institute which found that mouthwash was associated with cancer of the mouth and throat among women who neither smoked nor drank." [171]

In order to stop bad breath, it is necessary to oxidise the volatile sulphur compounds. Anthium dioxide has been found to do this safely and effectively. Mouthwashes containing this component are effective in helping control tooth decay and gum disease through their ability to oxidise and dissolve food films that cling to the teeth and build up on the gums. I recommend this type of mouthwash use twice a day, a capful at a time. I have a long distance lorry driver as a patient. I told him to use a capful to help him with his bleeding gums. He came back a week later for another bottle having finished this one in record time. On questioning, he revealed that he thought I said a cupful at a time!

SWEET AND SOUR?
Whilst in practice in Australia, I had a patient who had just consumed a Chinese take-away meal. I could smell this guy's breath while he was still in the waiting room. I decided that my stomach wasn't up to treating him, and so I gave him a bottle of stabilised chlorine dioxide mouthwash. He returned in one week with no bad breath at all!

CHLORHEXIDINE
Chlorhexidine is probably the most well known mouthwash used by the dental profession. In Sweden, it is the product of choice. It acts in three distinct ways:

- It disturbs the normal membrane functions of the bacteria, especially streptococcus mutans.

---

[171] Steinman, D and Epstein S, *Safe Shoppers Bible*, ibid.

- It interferes with adhesion of the bacteria to the tooth and pellicle by affecting a surface enzyme.
- It interferes with a glycolytic enzyme, which leads to a reduced acid production by the bacteria.

The side-effects of this product are mainly discolouration of teeth, teeth restorations, dentures and the tongue. It is quite common to have a black tongue within a week. It can also affect taste and cause soreness of the oral mucosa.

Chlorhexidine was always my mouthwash of choice for oral infections. However since trying a stabilised chlorine dioxide mouthwash, I have little use for any other as this product performs well.

FLOSS

It is difficult to get enthusiastic about floss. You either love it or you hate it! But it needs to get in between those teeth. The manufacturers do all sorts of things with it, including adding mint and fluoride to it.

There is nothing worse than having floss that frays. Like many dentists, I have had to remove frayed bits of floss from between teeth. Of course, if all fillings and crowns had perfect margins with no overhangs, then the fraying wouldn't be a problem. Occasionally when fillings are placed, they are packed so that they overhang the edge of the preparation. When the filling sets, there is a ledge that traps food and debris and snags on floss. The edge needs to be removed in order to be able to keep the area clean. So if you have snagging of floss, then you need to return to your dentist for help.

TONGUE SCRAPER

Some dentists recommend tongue scraping as anaerobic bacteria can reside in the deep fissures of the tongue.

TOOTHBRUSHES

They come in all shapes and sizes and with bristles going every which way. Marketing dictates that brushes need to be continuously re-invented. In 1977, I carried out research on patients suffering rheumatoid arthritis. I found that the electric toothbrush was most effective even compared to a toothbrush with an enlarged handle. There is no doubt that for special groups there is a need to modify the brush or use an electric one. Manual brushing still has its place and is effective if carried out correctly.

BRUSH UP ON YOUR BRUSHING

A new report says that two thirds of us aren't using our toothbrushes properly, even when we think we are. In the following article, Dr. James Steele, of Newcastle University Dental School, states:

"Although more people are flossing and using a mouthwash, their dental technique is wrong... Look for a brush with a narrow head that can easily reach all corners of the mouth and medium textured, tightly packed bristles that are rounded at the ends. A brush that is too hard won't scrub your teeth cleaner and may damage your gums." [172]

I like my patients to have a systematic brushing regime. Random brushing generally leads to an area being missed. Brush down over the gums, wriggle the bristles under the gum line and then scrub the biting surfaces of the teeth. Some dentists recommend dry brushing, followed by toothpaste. Others like flossing after brushing. Personally, I advise to floss before brushing and if needed again afterwards. This allows for debris to be dislodged and then removed with brushing.

AND THE CHEWING GUM
THAT MAKES TEETH HEALTHIER

The Daily Mail has just printed the following article on chewing gum:

"A toothpaste manufacturer has developed a chewing gum that fights decay and whitens teeth. It contains zinc acetate which combats the bacteria that cause bad breath and decay. It is a plaque inhibitor and fights the bacteria that cause bad breath. The

---

[172] *Daily Express*, 28th March, 2000

whitening gum has a low abrasive silica in it which gently cleans the teeth and rubs away tea and coffee stains." [173]

In the next chapter, I discuss treating people for jaw joint problems. Constant chewing can aggravate the symptoms in people who already have a jaw problem. While chewing non-toxic gum may help the teeth in certain circumstances, let caution be exercised in those with clicking jaws and with head or neck pain.

SUMMARY
Your dentist or hygienist is the best person to advise on technique. If it works, don't change it. If it doesn't, then seek advice.

Oral hygiene is not just about bad breath and tooth decay, it now encompasses your overall health. The use of good quality, non-harmful, toxin-free products, good technique, consistency and the right equipment is essential for good all-round health. Attention to nutrition and adequate water intake will only enhance results.

---

[173] UK *Daily Mail*, Tuesday, 14th August, 2001

A History of Pain

Amie is a mother of three and a self-employed dairy farmer. For thirty-two years she had but one ambition, to live her life without pain. So as not to detract from her experience, I have copied her letter in full, omitting only her full name, date of birth and address.

"Firstly, God bless Dr. Bill Read. When I was sent to this man by chiropractor, Dr. Michael Troy, I was more than sceptical, very angry, frustrated and sick of living my life as a chronic pain sufferer. I was a headache cripple, very weepy, depressed and anxious. I had lived with constant pain since I was 18 years old. Most times, I suffered shocking pain in my head, neck and back. Pain was my constant enemy and life was hell!

I'd rather not describe the days when I lived in bed, knocked out on useless drugs, vomiting and wishing I was game enough to commit suicide.

Early life
I had a normal, happy, country upbringing. At around 12 years of age, my teeth became mal-positioned with over-shot bottom teeth. I wore bands between the ages of 13 – 16. At aged 18, I had a bad fall from a racehorse. I lost my memory and I have never been able to remember what happened. My jaws and mouth have never felt comfortable. My jaws and teeth moved back after removal of the bands. I have always clenched my teeth – never ground.

At 21, the shocking headaches began, followed by all other pains. By 37, I suffered chronic pain all the time with every type of headache possible. I had months away in hospital, going to a chiropractor daily, including weekends. I could hardly walk, let alone work or be a mother.

I've seen nearly every type of doctor there is:

General Practitioner
Specialists
Neurologists
Psychologists
Psychiatrists
Acupuncturists
Chiropractors
Naturopaths
Physiotherapists
Etc. etc.

I've had nearly every test there is - blood tests, brain scans, eg. X-rays, revealing no brain tumours. Those wonderful men and women of medicine described me as:

Overworked
Overstressed
In need of a holiday
A worrier
Emotionally imbalanced
Manic depressive
A sufferer of every type of headache possible
Neurological pain
Shocking back
Bad neck
Ear pain

When Dr. Bill Read put the splint in my mouth – the pains started to subside within 12 hours and the migraines subsided in frequency and intensity. My general health improved greatly. The only pills I take now are Evening Primrose Oil. I'm still in a state of shock after 12 weeks – I can sometimes feel pain trying to start up in my head, but it does not seem to be able to get going. I am hardly game to take "my" bite plate out of my mouth, except to clean it.

Thank God for Dr. Bill Read and long may he do his work. I am grateful to him forever."

But I say, *"To Him be the glory and the dominion forever and ever. Amen."* (1 Peter 5: 11)

THE MOUTH IS A PART OF THE BODY

I couldn't finish this book without touching on the area of dentistry that has consumed my life for the last 16 years; pain that so often appears bizarre and baffling to the medical and dental professions; pain that has robbed people of their dreams, hopes and desires; pain that has broken marriages, destroyed lives and ruined businesses; pain that has no logical origin, explained away as *all in the head, overworked, stressed, depressed, hormonal* and many more unkind, untrue, sanctimonious comments that describe pain that is most likely dental in origin.

In 1985, I listened for the first time to a Dr Harold Gelb, DMD. This larger-than-life New York dentist would start his lectures thus:

"The mind is like a parachute; it only functions when open."

He was referring to the paradigm shift that dentists need to make in order to see the wider importance of the mouth as part of the body. Arguably, Harold's legacy was his ability to make dentists realise that the mouth is part of the whole.

In his book, *Killing Pain Without Prescription,* Dr Gelb writes:

"If you suffer from headache, neckache, backache or other chronic discomfort, you'll be tested for many diseases and disorders in an attempt to find the cause of the pain. You may be tested for all kinds of obscure afflictions, but ironically, you probably won't be checked for the most common purveyor of pain: TMJ syndrome." [174]

TMJ refers to the temporo-mandibular joint. This is the jaw joint. Gelb and other researchers found that misalignment of the jaw caused myriad symptoms that could be treated by the simple insertion of a dental splint. This is a piece of plastic, made to sit

---

[174] Gelb, H, & Paula M Seigel *Killing Pain Without Prescription*, Barnes & Noble, 1982

over the upper or lower teeth. It works by realigning the jaw and normalising function. It only works when in the mouth, as it is not an orthodontic appliance. It does not make permanent changes. This normalisation often brings quick relief from the muscular pain and stresses on the body caused by TMJ dysfunction.

NO ONE COULD HELP HER

Wendy says, *"My splint saved my life!"* Over twenty years ago she began to experience left-sided facial pain. This started as aches and pains in her teeth. Nothing was found on the X-ray, but the persistence of her pain led her dentist to root-fill the lower molars of the affected side. This produced no relief, whereupon the dentist decided that extraction was required. Her teeth were removed, but the pain still present. Wendy consulted her general medical practitioner who referred her to the specialist maxillo-facial unit. They knew what the problem was but couldn't treat it. She went back to the doctor who prescribed anti-depressants. She felt that this was the start of her long-term major depression. No one could help her. Her pain interfered with her lifestyle and challenged her relationship.

THAT'S ME!

Then she read *'Killing Pain Without Prescription'*. *"That's me!"* she exclaimed and phoned one of the references given in the back of the book. She was referred to a dentist with a special interest in TMJ. He fitted her with a Gelb splint. The pain didn't go immediately. But gradually, with adjustments of the splint and osteopathic care, her life became normal. No longer was she in pain, no longer did people label her as mad. No more was she going here, there and everywhere to find a solution. Now, twenty years later, she still wears a splint, which I occasionally adjust for her. She believes that this treatment has quite literally **saved her life.**

Since Gelb's early lectures I have encountered many different names for this phenomenon. TMJ is only one.

MANY NAMES, ONE CONDITION

Dr Aelred Fonder named this condition: 'Dental Distress Syndrome. (DDS)'

"Dental Distress Syndrome is the distress produced by mal-occluded teeth and the resultant spasms and malfunctioning of the musculature of the jaws, head, neck and shoulders, causing physio-pathological alterations throughout all the systems of the soma and psyche. Dental Distress routinely produces Selye's General Adaptation Syndrome.

Widespread normalisation is observed in all systems of soma and psyche, when a corrective dental splint restores occlusal balance, allowing the powerful muscles of mastication to function at their physiological contracting and resting lengths." [175]

This dental mal-occlusion routinely causes spinal mal-posturing, pelvic rotation, uneven shoulder height and head tilt. Removal of the excessive stress of dental origin allows posture to normalise.

Other names such as myofascial pain dysfunction syndrome and disorders of the functional occlusal system have been used to describe this condition. I am sure there are many more. So why did I have such a keen interest in this condition? Why did it capture my imagination? By way of explanation, let me tell my own story.

My patients would sometimes look at me and say, *"You don't know what it's like to live like this pain day after day, with no one really believing that there is anything wrong."* And I would look them straight in the eye and say: *"Oh, yes I do!"*

MY HEADACHE

It was 1985 when my headaches struck. I had been doing the unforgivable in headache terms. I was dieting (which for me was starvation), I was exercising and I was stressed out with my dental practice. Whilst at the gym, I attempted lifting a certain weight and I felt a tear on the left hand side of my neck. I ignored it and went home.

---

[175] Fonder, Aelred, Paper presented at the 2nd International Symposium on the Management of Stress, Monaco, 18th-22nd November 1977

RED HOT POKER IN THE EYE
Within 10 days, I was in hospital with the worst headache of my life. It started as a sharp shooting pain in my left eye that would awaken me at 3 am. I would swing my legs over the side of the bed and cry until the pain reduced twenty minutes later. Exhausted, I would sleep again. The next night it was the same and the next night and the next. I couldn't eat and I really felt that I was dying. Andy, my local doctor and rugby team-mate, came to visit me. Within a few hours I was in hospital. I stayed there for 3 weeks, having had a brain scan, numerous X-rays, a lumbar puncture, ergotamine treatment and a questionable diagnosis of viral encephalitis.

CLUSTER MIGRAINES
I left hospital with drug-induced double vision and weighing 2 stone lighter. At least I'd lost the weight, but unfortunately it was mainly from my legs, and I could hardly walk up the stairs. It was eight weeks before I returned to work. The diagnosis then changed from viral encephalitis to cluster migraine with a diagnosed threat of recurrence. My personal diagnosis was myofascial pain dysfunction brought on by the injury and stress. Here was a case of two different professions looking at the same problem from different points of view.

Having exhausted the medical model, they came up with a dubious diagnosis based on their knowledge. From a dental perspective there were options that were not available to the doctors. In my case, it was the dental model that proved affective. To treat my condition, I turned to a dentist for help.

TREATMENT
My teeth were built up to the correct height of the bite, using composite filling material. This was carried out initially by Dr Fonder. Chiropractic and osteopathic care was instigated with the result of no more pain! And even today, if I let the bite height wear down, the pain returns.

There is little doubt that occlusal disorders have a profound affect on the rest of the body. This is not so strange when it is realised that somewhere between 30 and 50 percent of the total sensory and motor input is from the head and neck. This is a lot of bytes on your human computer.

I tell my own story as one of hope to those people who have been everywhere and done everything except seek the advice of a dentist trained in head and neck pain of dental origin.

PAIN DEFIED DESCRIPTION
At 70, Betty lived a full and active life. Then for no apparent reason, she started to suffer head pains. For three years there was no relief, day or night from this relentless pain. It was a pain that would start at the base of the skull and spread over the head and into the temples – a pain that defied description or location. Tension headaches, she would call them, headaches that could grow into a full-blown migraine, with facial numbness and flashing lights. She had a history of nocturnal tooth-grinding and tinnitus (ringing in the ears)/vertigo which had started in 1976.

PAIN GONE IN 24 HOURS
Chiropractic had helped to relieve her symptoms somewhat, but nothing really shifted the pain. A brain scan was ordered to find the elusive cause, but nothing was found. Medication was prescribed which only made her sleepy and less able to function on a daily basis. Her chiropractor referred her to me as she felt that the problem was jaw-related. After examination, I agreed and fitted her with a night-time splint. Her pain went within 24 hours and has not returned.

IN PAIN FOR 19 YEARS
Heather had 19 years of pain. At the age of 13, she had teeth removed for orthodontic reasons. She suffered with buckteeth. Her dentist then proceeded to push all of her teeth back to correct her bite. The treatment went on for quite a while and the dentist became unsure of his ability to complete the task and achieve a satisfactory result. He referred her to hospital for a consultant's opinion. They said that the treatment had gone wrong and that she would require surgery to repair the damage. This would involve major surgery to the jaws, both of which would need to be broken and moved to the correct position. This would also reshape the face.

The success rate for this operation was estimated at 40%. Her father had declined the surgery on her behalf.

From the age of 20, she began to suffer pains in her shoulder and back. She couldn't stand for long periods of time or bend to do the gardening. She was diagnosed with tendonitis and injected with steroids.

She was seen by one of my colleagues who was concerned about her worn-down teeth and he referred her to me. By this time, the back and neck pain had developed into headaches. I fitted her with a dental splint at the correct bite height and the pain reduced. Within a couple of weeks the pain had disappeared and has not returned. She is pleased and her GP is amazed!

COULD I HELP LAURIE?
I saw Laurie today. This beautiful young lady was suffering from bilateral repetitive strain injury in her arms. A computer operator and phone receptionist, she would spend her days typing and crooking the phone between her shoulder and the side of her head. She started to experience headaches, severe neck pain and pain in the arms. Physiotherapy and wrist splints were recommended to help with the pain and function. She thought that the pain was worse since the wrist supports had been fitted.

On questioning, she said that she had had extraction orthodontics with the removal of four first premolars. The result didn't look too bad, but the lower jaw had been driven back by the procedure causing a forward head posture and compression of the cervical spine. I palpated her neck and back which were both really sore. I then advanced the lower jaw and repalpated. The pain went instantly. Treatment will be aimed at correcting the lower jaw position and osteopathy to help with the neck and back problem. The diagnosis and treatment that Laurie had been given was inappropriate for her condition. How many Lauries are out there suffering through lack of knowledge?

PROFESSIONAL DEBATE OR PRIDE
Tooth extraction for orthodontic reasons is a hotly disputed subject. The debate is whether extraction ruins facial outline. It

would appear that facial appearance is only one problem. Changing the relationship of the teeth to each other and to the TMJ affects the cervical spine.

According to Guzay, the pivotal point of rotation of the jaw is between the first two vertebrae. [176] This effectively means that if the jaw joint goes into dysfunction, there will be a compensation and dysfunction of the cervical spine also. While the changes occur at cervical spines C1 and C2, the pathology is often seen on X-ray lower down the cervical spine with degeneration commonly occurring at C4, C5, and C6. So the change that occurred due to extraction in Laurie's case may well have brought about the pathology she was now experiencing. All in the search for beauty. What a price to pay!

While the teeth are straight at the end of treatment, they often relapse by the age of 21, with re-crowding of the lower front teeth. The face seldom improves, but often appears to have been damaged. The patient adopts a forward head posture and head, neck and back pain ensues.

The shame is that Gelb and others have given us a template for examination criteria that could help us prevent these problems before they arise. It is quite simple to examine a child and find out what problems they already have. If they suffer headaches and neck pain before tooth removal, then it would be better not to go ahead with extraction and train tracks. It would be preferable to expand the jaws and allow growth to do its own thing. This is functional orthodontics and makes for common sense. What is not common sense is to treat a growing child without knowing what is going on in the rest of the body.

ACCIDENTS HAPPEN

A few years ago, a lady was referred to me by her orthopaedic surgeon. She was suffering a great deal of dental pain and was having difficulty opening her mouth. She had been playing the

---

[176] Guzay, C M, "Quadrant Theorem", 1952. This paper is available by contacting Credence Publications, PO Box 3, Tonbridge, Kent. TN12 9ZY, UK (www.credence.org)

organ in church and on reaching a crescendo up the top end, she fell off the organ stool and damaged her hip. She was taken to hospital where she was treated for the resultant hip and back problem. While these were being treated, she developed tooth pain on the right side of her face.

DEAD TEETH

She visited her dentist who decided that one of her teeth had died and set about doing a root canal. Once this was completed, she still had the pain. He root-filled another, then another. Having root-filled three of the teeth in the upper jaw, the pain was still there. He then root-filled the three opposing teeth in the lower jaw. The pain persisted and the patient, believing that this dentist was no good, sought a second opinion. The second dentist redid all of the work and yet the pain persisted. The result was that all six teeth were removed and the pain persisted. After all of this, the patient was sent to me.

On questioning her more closely, I discovered that, in falling from the stool, she had hit her jaw on the keyboard. On examination, there was limited jaw opening with pain and discomfort in the joints and the musculature of the cheeks and sides of the head. I decided to fit splint dentures to correct the problem and relieve her pain.

In the *Trigger Point Manual*, Janet Travell, MD demonstrated that not all toothache comes from the teeth. Some of it comes from the muscles and trigger points within the head and neck.[177] The temporalis muscle, which is on the side of the head above the ear, gives rise to pain that mimics toothache in the upper back teeth. The anterior belly of the digastric, which sits under the front of the chin, gives pain in the lower front teeth. If this is not known, then these teeth will be treated without looking for the possibility that the muscle is the problem.

---

[177] Travell, J G & D G Simons "Myofascial Pain and Dysfunction", *The Trigger Point Manual*, Williams & Wilkins, 1983

WHEN PAIN IS NOT WHAT IT APPEARS TO BE

This was what happened to the organist. Her problem was not dental but muscular. Now, before we give the dentist a hard time, it is difficult to convince a person that their pain is not what they think it is!

A lady came to see me who suffered daily headaches for years. Every morning, her children would make her a cup of tea and let her lay in bed, in the hope that the headache would lift. She came to see me with a poorly fitting upper denture and a few lower teeth, including one in the back on the lower right side. I built up the lower back tooth with composite white filling material and she was pain-free in less than 24 hours.

PSYCHIATRIST OR DENTIST?

Many of the patients that I see have been everywhere, done everything and nothing had worked. They are eventually shipped off to the psychiatrist or pain management consultant when all they needed was a dentist.

THE IMPORTANCE OF THE BITE

The intricacy of the bite has never really been fully evaluated. Teeth or no teeth, we seem to function. If it hurts, pull it out; a few teeth more or less - what's the difference? When I was first in practice, it was quite common to extract a tooth and leave a gap, especially under the terms of the health service where there was no mandatory requirement to replace the missing tooth, so long as the patient could be deemed dentally fit. For the most part people continue to function, and after a relatively short period of time, they become used to the space.

IT'S ALL A QUESTION OF BALANCE

Imagine you have to have your foot removed. No one offers you anything to replace it. Every time you stand up you fall over. Why? It's a matter of balance. You know that if you get a stone in your shoe or have a sore foot, the next thing you get is backache. You have teeth removed on one side of your jaw with no replacement, and the next thing you know, you are suffering from headaches and neck pain. It's all a matter of balance.

It makes sense when you think about it, and yet there are numerous people suffering needlessly because no one has bothered to replace the missing teeth and effect balance within the mouth.

DENTAL SPLINTS
Dental splints or dentures give this balance. They replace the missing teeth, restore the loss of bite height and help change the jaw-to-jaw relationship. Once fitted and adjusted, they put the mouth and jaws back into balance. This balance helps generally to stabilise the body. Unfortunately, this is not always looked for, as we shall see.

CONVENTION OR ENTRENCHED ERROR?
The criteria within which we work as dentists is to look at the teeth, gums and supporting tissues, with little regard for the rest of the body. For example:

A young girl attends with dental crowding, *"Daddy's teeth, Mummy's jaws."* The whole family want her to look great but at the moment she has buck-teeth and is called 'Bugs Bunny' at school. The line of treatment offered is extraction of four teeth and braces to reduce the crowding and align the teeth. Two years later she has a great looking set of teeth, sitting in a mouth that's too small, with no chin and an unhappy, strained look. Further investigation reveals that prior to treatment, she had suffered head and neck pain, earache and a curved spine. Since treatment, the headaches have become more severe, the jaw joints now lock and the back pain has increased. She also suffers from painful periods, has an irritable bowel, poor concentration and has just contracted chronic fatigue syndrome or ME.

THE ALTERNATIVE
The girl's treatment could have gone as follows: the dentist notes crowded teeth accompanied by head and neck pain: on analysis of the posture, the spinal curvature is noted and referral is made to the chiropractor, where it is found that she has a leg length discrepancy and flat feet. Referral to a podiatrist would see her recommended orthotics for her shoes, ongoing chiropractic care for her postural problems and then back to the dentist. Instead of tooth-removal, expansion of the deficient jaws would take place,

using orthopaedic appliances with screws in them to expand the jaws: this would result in wide smiles, good cheek bones, good-looking faces and reduction in symptoms, with every chance that these will not return.

You can take your pick if you can afford to pay! Under general National Health Service terms in the UK, these treatments are not usually available.

WHAT ABOUT THE CHILDREN?

Jane came to us suffering blinding headaches. The pain was so bad that she was constantly off school, lying in a darkened air-conditioned room, regularly swallowing painkillers, drifting in and out of sleep, hoping that, upon waking, somehow the pain would have gone.

According to her mother, Jane had lost a lot of weight. Generally a healthy, happy child, she had become reclusive and quiet, no longer wishing to join in the fun and games or spend time with the family. She was desperate, her mother was desperate and we were the last glimmer of hope for this family who had begged the orthodontist to remove the braces that were ruining her life.

ETHICS OR MORAL OBLIGATION?

Ethics dictated that we should not intervene. Though Jane's mother insisted and our hearts ached for this girl, there was nothing we could do. The orthodontist was the specialist. Apparently he knew what he was doing. He had commenced the treatment and it was not right that we meddle in his affairs.

After our advice that she should once again return to the orthodontist in question, she left the practice dismayed. Her last glimmer of hope was now a dying ember. She did indeed return to the orthodontist who said that the treatment had nothing to do with the head pain and that she should see her medical doctor for these. He was just straightening her teeth. The doctor found nothing medically wrong and so another frantic, pleading phone call to our practice was made – a call we could no longer ignore.

NO ONE DESERVES TO LIVE LIKE THIS

No one deserved to go through this just to have straight teeth. Jane was given an appointment and, with the consent of her parents, the fixed braces were removed. Within 24 hours, the pain had gone and soon Jane was able to get back to the life that had been denied her for so long. There followed a brief spell of dental politics, various mud slinging meetings and an eventual apology on our part to the orthodontist for interfering in 'specialist' work. We had interfered with the wheels of the dental machine, but Jane was ecstatic and her mum was over the moon. I believe we did exactly what needed to be done.

Now don't get me wrong, I do actually have some really good friends who are orthodontists doing amazing work and obtaining great results. However, the end doesn't always justify the means, especially when the end may bring residual headaches, neck pain, ringing in the ears and clicking jaws - not to mention the relapse or re-crowding that can occur unless long-term retention is used.

We expose our teeth to sugar, fluoride, amalgam fillings and then remove them from their overcrowded, little jaws - all by the tender age of 12 or 13. *"Mummy's jaws, Daddy's teeth."* I hear you say. *"She's got her father's teeth. They're really too big for her mouth. And you can see that she has inherited my jaws. They took out some teeth to make room to move and straightened the rest so that she would have straight teeth and a beautiful smile."*

The trouble is that while the orthodontist has produced a beautiful set of straight gnashers minus four, the faces are often less than attractive. The head and neck are leaning forward with resultant head and neck pain, clicking, locking jaws and an uptight teenager. What could follow that? A diagnosis of ADD maybe and a prescription for Ritalin?

NO MISTAKE

At the risk of sounding pious, God didn't get it wrong. If He built us with 32 teeth, then the chances are that 32 is the number He wanted. So if He didn't make a mistake, what has happened that we should demand extractions for our kids and appliances to make them beautiful?

Dr Weston Price had found the answer:

"The physiques of the primitive Indians of the far north who were still living in their isolated locations and in accordance with their accumulated wisdom were superb. There were practically no irregular teeth, including no impacted third molars, as evidenced by the fact that all individuals old enough to have the molars erupted had them standing in position and functioning normally for mastication." [178]

Where the Indians were using white man's food, tooth decay was severe and they developed crooked teeth with deformed dental arches.

QUALITY REPLACED BY QUANTITY

Dr Price's research found tribes with excellent teeth while most of the 'civilised' populations today possess wretched teeth. There is no doubt in my mind that we have paid a high price for chemicalising and denaturing our food so that it will not rot on the shelf (quality replaced by quantity). Have we not attractively packaged our tasteless fruits and vegetables to better appeal to the unsuspecting and undeserving public?

With our teeth, we have a skeletal problem. Poor nutrition leads to poor growth. Europeans have understood this for years but, rather than resort to good nutrition as a base, they have partially treated the problem with functional appliances. These are removable orthopaedic appliances that work with the growth of the child in an attempt, if you like, to catch up with the growth that has not occurred. But is it not better to sort out the basics? Fonder states that:

"Removable appliance therapy is rapidly gaining favour in America after years of rejection by their orthodontists." [179]

---

[178] Price, Weston A, ibid.
[179] Fonder, Aelred, ibid.

ALIGN, ROTATE, UPRIGHT AND TORQUE

Europeans, after years of functional appliance utilisation, are beginning to favour fixed appliances. What both groups should be discovering is that skeletal problems respond best to functional appliances while ideal case finishing is best accomplished through banding or bonding brackets to align, rotate, upright and torque the teeth. Functional appliances cannot achieve this exacting tooth positioning. So dentists of the world, unite! There's room for us all to work side by side here.

Extracting teeth and collapsing the dental arches can lock the cranial bones, causing displeasing relationships between the teeth, leading to facial bone malformation, bite and postural problems. For this reason, we are seeing a process of rethinking and the American acceptance of functional orthopaedic appliances.

A great teacher and friend of mine, Dr Dick Pertes of the University of Medicine and Dentistry, New Jersey, once said:

"If the only tool you have is a hammer, you see every problem as a nail."

Dick was head of the TMJ program at the University and a past orthodontist who realised that he needed more than a hammer to sort out the problems he was seeing in practice. The difficulty is one of diagnosis and then having the tools for the job.

Orthodontics – Another Health War

When I first started looking at headaches, I was just looking at adults. These were people who had lost teeth through neglect, decay or trauma and others who had always looked after their teeth but their gnashers were worn due to constant grinding or clenching that produced tooth fracture and loss of bite height. I also saw people who suffered jaw pain with locking of the joint, head, neck and back pain of muscular origin due to changes in the bite; people who, as the result of extractions, had over-eruption of the other teeth, causing premature contacts and dental interferences that led to myofascial pain dysfunction syndrome.[180]

This was my introduction to the study of TMJ disorders. As time went by, another group emerged that would appear to have an iatrogenic causation - post-orthodontic cases. These people were suffering head, neck and back pain, locking of the jaws, wear of the lower teeth, tightening of the lips and cheeks, forward head posture and generalised pains throughout the body. These people were being treated dentally for a skeletal problem.

STRAIGHT TEETH
We have come to understand orthodontics as a means of straightening crooked teeth. If there are too many teeth, then usually four first premolars are extracted and the remaining teeth are aligned, using fixed braces and sometimes headgear for extra anchorage to pull the teeth into place. This tends to pull the teeth and face backwards which, according to Enlow, is opposite to growth, which is essentially forward.[181]

This concept is picked up by Gelb who treated TMJ cases with appliances that bring the lower jaw down and forward to relieve pain and normalise the relationship between the upper jaw, lower jaw and the cervical spine.[182] The cause of Jane's pain was that her

---

[180] Travell, J G & D Simons, ibid.
[181] Enlow, D H *Facial Growth*, W B Saunders Company, Harcourt Brace Jovanovich Inc., 1990
[182] Gelb, Harold *Clinical Management of Head, Neck and TMJ Pain and Dysfunction*, W B Saunders & Company, 1985

jaw wanted to grow down and forward while the orthodontist wanted to pull her up and back. Not satisfied with preventing her growing in the intended direction, he was attempting to pull her back in the opposite direction.

OPPOSING FORCES

For those of you who wonder why some fixed orthodontics go on forever, the answer is that there are two opposing forces fighting for direction. Each time the braces are removed, the growth tendency is to move forward again, the teeth re-crowd until finally, in desperation, a fixed retainer is stuck onto the teeth to hold them in place. If this is not enough, then headgear with whiskers (a wire attached to the appliance that pokes out of the mouth like a cat's whisker) can be used to give more anchorage and backward pulling power. X-rays show that when cervical traction is used, it can detrimentally affect the neck, increasing the curvature of the cervical spine and thus initiating the onset of headaches by compressing the posterior neck muscles.

By the age of 21, the teeth start to kink and re-crowd. Enter the oral surgeon, knife in hand, ready to remove the wisdom teeth that supposedly cause this late onset crowding. Now we have eight teeth on the floor rather than four, and the problem is still there. What I see in practice is crowding and, in certain cases, the onset of the symptoms described before.

WHY THE PERFECT SMILE
COULD RUIN YOUR HEALTH

According to Marion McKay of the Daily Mail, more parents than ever before are encouraging their children to put braces on their teeth in an effort to give them the perfect smile – but it's a practice that many believe could lead to a lifetime of back pain, headaches and sore limbs. According to some in the industry, far from enhancing children's profiles, these methods can lead to longer, flatter faces, prolonged damage to the skull and cause headaches, jaw and muscle pain.[183] Dr John Mew, an outspoken

---

[183] "Why The Perfect Smile Could Ruin Your Health", *Daily Mail*, November 30, 1999

critic of the trend for extracting teeth and applying fixed braces, says:

> *"I frequently see examples of faces which have been really badly spoiled. In my opinion, probably about 20% of orthodontic patients are noticeably damaged and maybe another 30% are slightly damaged."* [184]

Critics say that by extracting teeth in the top of the mouth and pulling back others to match the bottom teeth, the lower jaw is effectively locked in. This prevents the lower jaw growing forwards properly. The resultant symptoms were described earlier in the previous chapter.

PROBLEMS WITH THE UPPER RUNG

If we are not going to extract the teeth, what can be done? Dr Mew has his own set of appliances that are used to expand the upper jaw and then align the lower jaw to the upper. This is on the understanding that the problem is one of a small upper jaw or maxilla. The appliances are then expanded to aid growth of the upper jaw. Most of them have some sort of screw, which is turned by the patient on a daily or weekly basis. This turning slowly expands the bones of the upper jaw in an attempt to achieve a more normal maxillary size. Once this has been achieved, the lower jaw is advanced and a balance obtained between the upper and lower jaw and teeth. This balance helps to normalise the relationship between the teeth, jaw joints and the cervical spine. This aids in uprighting the head on the neck and allows normal function of the spine.

FUNCTIONAL APPLIANCES

John Mew is not alone in his endeavour. As with many things dental, there are a variety of appliances. Some bear the name of the inventor, such as Frankel, Schwartz, Clarke or with names like Bionator, Biobloc and the new ALF light wire removable appliance system that has done away with the bulky size of the older appliances but not their effectiveness.

---

[184] Dr John Mew is the Clinical Director of The London School of Facial Orthotropics, Surrey, UK. He lectures worldwide on the orthotropic premise.

The range of techniques offered has caused some disturbance within the orthodox orthodontic community. Entrenched beliefs have been challenged. Research has been put forward on both sides which has only polarised opinion.

Dr Noel Stimson, editor of *Cranio-View*, a UK-based journal of the Cranio Group and the Society for the Study of Cranio-Mandibular Disorders, has this to say about a recent Channel 4 *Dispatches* TV program on the orthodontic dispute:

"I found it quite depressing that the 'seniors' in the orthodontic establishment should display such studied ignorance – deliberate head-in-the-sand stuff. What does it take to get them to wake up to the reality that some kids' faces are being ruined by orthodontic expediency? Taking refuge behind a skewed view of the 'evidence' is unacceptable and does no credit to the orthodontic profession. This refers to two of the most experienced and respected orthodontic specialists actually denying that extraction orthodontics has even the potential for damaging children's faces."[185]

BLIND RESEARCHERS
The problem revolves around research. The functional orthodontists depend on research and what is called anecdotal evidence - what they see with their own eyes. The academics on the other hand only believe the research. Noel says that he was horrified. Are they totally incapable of believing their own eyes unless there is "scientific evidence" to back it up? Have they not read the studies by Stellzig (1999) or Melson (1999) to name but two? Are they seriously suggesting that even a small number of anecdotal cases have no validity? Might they sit up and take notice only when there are significant numbers of facially-damaged children?

WARFARE
Once again the battle rages, but what of the patients? Dr Robert Walker is a chiropractor who has done a great deal of work in putting the whole picture together. The problem we dentists were

---

[185] Stimson, Noel, *View Point*, Cranio-View, Island Printers, Isle of Wight, 1999

having was understanding why the things we were seeing in the mouth had such an effect on the rest of the body. We were also unsure about what to treat first. All the time we were just straightening teeth, we were fulfilling our remit and there was no problem. Then we realised that problems were occurring that needed answers.

As dentists we were not aware of the relationship between the mouth and the rest of the body. Drs Gelb, Fonder, Stack and Farrar helped to take us out of the mouth and show us that what we were doing directly impacted the rest of the body. What we needed to know was when the problem started in the mouth and when in the body.

CHIRODONTICS
Dr Walker came to the rescue and found the missing link - how to discern the origin of the skeletal problem. Once we knew this, we could work out a treatment plan that could help the whole body. Bob has called this Chirodontics.

If the dental profession as a whole adopted his system, fewer children would be damaged. Patient assessment would enable us to discern who has skeletal problems before treatment commences. Who already suffers head, neck and back pain? Who can go straight to orthodontics and who needs the chiropractor, osteopath or physiotherapist first?

Many people have had conventional orthodontics and are very happy with the result. They encounter no pain and no obvious damage as a result of the treatment. This chapter is not aimed at them, but at those who have spent their adult life in pain and misery. Selye said, that:

"Stress is the non-specific reaction of the body to any demand placed upon it. Stress also is cumulative." [186]

When we look at this from an orthodontic standpoint, we can consider the physical and emotional stress of having four teeth

---

[186] Selye, H, *Stress Without Distress*, ibid.

removed on the child - perhaps their first experience of treatment at the hand of the dentist. Up until this time, there had been no need for fillings or any other treatment. Now, as the result of crowding, the day comes for extraction. The child has no idea what is to come, other than horror stories from friends at school, feeding his imagination.

QUEST FOR BEAUTY

The needle, all 30mm of it, looks like the barrel of a twelve bore shotgun. It shoots a searing, burning slug of lignocaine with adrenaline straight into the soft tissues. The heart hardly has time to recover from the stabbing pain of the needle before the adrenaline hits again. The heart pumps so hard there's a definite possibility that it's going to pop straight out of the chest and land on the dentist's lap. This is what we put our children through in our quest for their beauty.

The structural stress is often apparent from an early age. Kyphoscoliotic patterns (spinal changes) become evident, dipped shoulders, a tipped pelvis, forward head posture, thru-the-mouth-breathing, sinus congestion, glue ear and headaches are evidence of pre-orthodontic correction. According to his theory of the 'tropic premise', John Mew believes that the teeth should be together and tongue should sit on the roof of the mouth 30-50% of the time, in order that good growth might occur.

EAR PROBLEMS

This is not the case in the forward-headed, thru-the-mouth breather, going for his fourth appointment for grommets. The removal of teeth and further embarrassment of the airway may well harm this child. The palate, already under-grown, is further compromised by extraction and reduction in the size of the dental arch. The result will be straight teeth, but ailing health will deteriorate further as the structural stresses accumulate. This child then goes from an uncomfortable childhood to pain throughout adult life.

It is imperative that a common examination procedure takes place which incorporates the whole body and not just the mouth. Diagnosis by looking at plaster casts, without looking at the patient must cease. Each case should be carefully weighed up to make sure that no harm is done to the child.

MILK OR WATER?

Many of the conditions I have seen over the years include nutritional deficiency. These children are often allergy-prone, with asthma, post-nasal drip, enlarged adenoids and an open mouth-breathing pattern. Treatment should include the removal of dairy from the diet. It must also include drinking lots of water. Dr Batmanghelidj emphasises the need for water and blames many of the western metabolic disease states on dehydration. Many children will reach for a bottle of milk, lemonade or coke in preference to water. According to this doctor, we need to re-hydrate. He says of the mouth:

"At the moment, a dry mouth is the only accepted sign of dehydration of the body. As I have explained, this signal is the last outward sign of extreme dehydration. The damage occurs at a level of persistent dehydration that does not necessarily demonstrate a dry mouth signal." [187]

DESTROYING LIVES

These children have major structural stressors and a reduced physiological range of adaptation. It doesn't take much to tip them over the edge from 'not sick' to 'sick'. If extraction orthodontics has to take place, then let it happen to the patient with a good immune system, a good adaptive range and an ability to cope with the emotional onslaught. It is imperative that the criteria for treatment be modified. No longer can we accept that the teeth are separate from the whole. No longer can we look at the teeth in isolation. No longer can we balance the bite without looking at the structural integrity of the whole system and no longer can we ignore the serious structural, emotional and chemical imbalances that are blighting our children and destroying their lives.

FRANCINE

This letter was written by Francine's mother:

---

[185] Batmanghelidj, F, *Your Body's Many Cries for Water*, ibid.

"We first brought Francine to Dr Read in 1989, when she was 8 years and 3 months, and had been suffering from vertigo for 18 months. For the last 3 months she also suffered ringing and roaring noise in her ears.

At that stage the vertigo attacks would occur at least once a week, maybe twice and last from one to three days at a time. During that time she would lay flat on her back and be unable to lift her head, walk without support or eat. Sometimes she experienced the top half of the world spinning in one direction and the bottom half in the opposite direction. Between attacks, she was always unsteady and would spend the day at school sitting in a bean bag chair, unable to sit or walk properly because of the dizziness.

The noises in her ears ranged from "soft" (and bearable) to "sounding like an aircraft taking off." She was withdrawn and constantly tense, with dark circles under her eyes. It seemed that perhaps it was sometimes related to some foods and on a naturopath's advice, we had removed dairy, citrus, chocolate and artificial colours/flavourings from her diet. However, the attacks continued.

VERTIGO
The vertigo attacks began in March 1988. By late November, the vertigo had become more severe. We went to the doctor who said it was probably viral.

By late January 1989, the vertigo had become distressing. We returned to the doctor, who ordered a CAT scan which showed nothing suspicious. We visited an ENT specialist who told us it was benign recurrent vertigo and that she would have to live with it. We took her to a naturopath who referred us to a chiropractor. We visited the chiropractor twice, but the vertigo continued. We tried another GP and a physiotherapist – whose initial treatment for a week seemed to bring some relief. But the vertigo continued.

Desperate, we returned to the ENT specialist, insisting that something be done. He ordered vestibular function test and an EEG – both of which produced normal results. He then referred us

147

to a paediatric neurologist, who finally decided Fran was suffering a form of migraine. He prescribed periactin, which, although it did dull the effects of the vertigo, left her feeling groggy and ravenously hungry.

A SPIN IN THE DENTIST'S CHAIR

Through a friend's recommendation we found our way to Dr Read in September 1989. After examining Fran, he put build-ups on her back teeth to open her bite, and within 20 minutes, the vertigo had subsided, and she was able to walk normally, and even spin on the dentist's chair – her head had become so steady. As the build-ups wore down, the vertigo returned. If they were too high, within 12 hours the vertigo returned. Eventually however, her head stabilised, so that by January 1990 the height of the build-ups was not a crucial issue.

During the next few months, with physiotherapy treatment, Fran broke her thumb-sucking and nail-biting habits and developed an attitude of readiness to wear the appliances necessary to correct her bite and hopefully prevent any further recurrence of the vertigo attacks.

Post Script:

By the time Fran commenced wearing appliances, the vertigo had almost completely disappeared. It returned only when swimming backstroke or butterfly, doing certain gymnastic movements and sometimes in connection with travel sickness, from which she suffers frequently.

However, just this month (March 1991), Fran swam both butterfly and backstroke in the school swimming carnival and gained a placing in both. It seemed to be a final statement on the success of the treatment being used, and a personal victory for her. Her confidence in her motor skills and movement in general is now fully restored, and we are very grateful."

FROM COLLAPSING BITE TO INSTANT FACELIFT

Fran's bite was a major factor in her life. Treatment saw great success and relief for the whole family. Collapsed bites can cause severe problems for many. We've all seen people whose chin almost touches their nose, who look as if they have no teeth and have wrinkles on their wrinkles. They use face creams, face paint and consider plastic surgery but no one looks for the answer inside the mouth. There you find ground down teeth, missing teeth, tilted teeth or wobbly, splaying teeth. The bite has collapsed. Restore the bite, remove the headaches, iron out the wrinkles and, hey Presto! An instant face-lift. No surgery involved!

TOM

Tom is a young lad from New South Wales who came to see me, suffering from a constant runny nose with obligatory green candlesticks hanging from each nostril, a narrow face, a mouth-breather and with forward-head posture. Orthodontic treatment was aimed at increasing the size of the upper jaw, thus opening up the sinuses, bringing the lower jaw forward, encouraging a change in the breathing habit and physiotherapy for the posture.

OOPS!

At the end of the consultation I discussed withdrawing dairy produce from his diet. I explained that often there is a lactose intolerance that perpetuates this problem and that his mother should instigate this for a period of three weeks. Sound advice, I thought. And silently, I congratulated myself for being so clever. The mother on the other hand gave me a look that could kill, gathered up her eight-year-old and marched out of the surgery. What had I done? I turned to my nurse for some reassurance, just a glimmer of a smile would have been sufficient. I was met with the same frozen look. This just wasn't my day. I had come to this little town to do some orthodontics and they must have been anti-British!

"Okay, what did I do?" I asked sheepishly, fearing an angry reply. The look turned to laughter as my nurse replied," *You don't know, do you? You really don't know!"* she squealed. *"They own one of the largest dairy farms in the whole of Northern New South Wales and you told them that milk is no good!"* Needless to say, they never came back. I wonder whether he still drinks milk?

THE NUTRITION CONNECTION

Research carried out by Dr Weston Price on primitive tribes living on a natural diet saw a change in dental and health status when these people changed to the western diet of refined sugar and white flour. He witnessed siblings of the same generation where the eldest child, fed on the indigenous diet, had wide jaws, no dental crowding or decay and suffered no ill-health. The child fed on the western diet had narrow jaws, dental crowding, decay and suffered ill-health.

"Dr Price studied numerous tribes of 14 different races all over the world. Invariably, no matter what their native diets or where they lived, these people had excellent teeth, extremely low decay rates, very little if any crookedness of teeth, and no impacted teeth. Most were magnificent specimens of health, with few illnesses, physical or mental." [188]

When these same people came in contact with our civilisation through the establishment of trading posts, etc., rampant tooth decay took place and first generation children developed severe crookedness of teeth and many of the same diseases and many other malformations exhibited in modern civilisation including cleft palates, harelips and club feet.

The items that so-called primitives received in trade were much the same everywhere; white flour and sugar. No matter where in the world these people lived, ninety percent of the total items they received in trade consisted of white flour and sugar. These two foods accounted for their severe degeneration and downfall.

DESTRUCTION OF THE ABORIGINES

Amongst the tribes researched by Weston Price were the Aborigines of Australia. Aborigines constitute a unique race. Price found them to be amongst the finest specimen of man, with superb eyesight, great health and hunting skills. [189] The growing boys were taught deference and esteem for their elders in a most impressive

---

[188] Fonder, Aelred, Medical & Dental Arts, 303 West 2nd St. Rock Falls, Illinois, 61071, USA
[189] Fonder, Aelred, Medical-Dental Arts, ibid.

way. This health and lifestyle has given way to poor nutrition, substance abuse and alcohol, for which they have little tolerance. Modern man has decimated this once fine race.

WE'RE STARVING TO DEATH

Who are we trying to kid? The research is stacked up against us; we are dying of diseases for which we are responsible. Heart disease is still the number one killer, cancer is at number two and iatrogenic (doctor-induced) illness and death is at number three.[190] To this we must add the killer of a poor western diet. I am a product of this system just as you are and it's not easy to find good food nowadays. The speed of our lives is such that fast food, fast cars and fast computers outstrip our physiological ability to cope. As a nation and as a society, we are stressed out, living in the fast lane and starving to death!

---

[190] Day, Phillip, *Health Wars*, ibid.

Snoring? Who's Snoring?

I'm Not Even Asleep Yet!

Half-way between sleep and consciousness, you hear a sound like roaring thunder. Sudden, sharp and ear-piercing, you realise that the sound is coming from your partner's mouth.

Snoring can make nervous wrecks out of even the most stalwart. Snoring can awaken the whole household with its intensity and vibration. Snoring has sent many a man to the spare room and many a women in desperation to seek help or solace from friends who suffer a similar existence.

You fall asleep and then the snoring starts again, louder this time, more frightening, more irritating, more violent. You try to settle your partner; a dig to the ribs, a kick to the shin, anything to stop the noise and allow you to fall into the now fitful sleep that has become the nightly pattern.

The snoring stops and so does the breathing. Now you're awake, your partner has stopped breathing. Maybe the kick was too hard? You wait, holding your breath for what seems an eternity, then with a sudden heave of the chest, a rasping, gasping for breath, the machine kicks back into action and it starts all over again. With the morning, your partner rises relatively refreshed and with no understanding of the torment that you have been through. They say, *"I can't believe that you want an extra half an hour in bed. You should have come to bed earlier!"*

BLEARY-EYED

Recently I was discussing snoring with a patient of mine. Her sleep had been disrupted to the point where she had banned her husband from the bedroom, and he ended up sleeping in the spare room. Not a good recipe for marriage and demoralising for the man who had no control over this problem. He came to see me for advice. He was in his forties, healthy, not overweight but with a jaw-to-jaw discrepancy, the lower jaw being well behind the upper, giving him a "buck tooth" appearance. I decided to treat him with a pull-forward appliance, to bring his lower jaw forward and thus open up his airway. I am pleased to say that he is now back in the matrimonial bed and both he and his wife sleep well. He is free from the noisy snoring that had kept her awake and severely tested their marriage.

HABITUAL SNORERS

Estimates vary as to the number of people who snore. BUPA states that snoring effects 45 percent of the population from time to time and that an estimated 25 percent of people are habitual snorers.[191] Epidemiological studies would suggest that just over 40% of middle-aged men snore and 30% of middle-aged women.[192]

Chambers Dictionary describes snoring as: *"Breathing roughly and hoarsely in sleep with vibration of the palate or the vocal chords, uvula and soft tissue."* [193] BUPA describes it as *'noisy breathing through the mouth and nose during sleep.'* It can occur when you are breathing in or out. Snoring occurs when air does not flow smoothly through the air passages, or when the soft tissues or muscles of the air passages vibrate. As you fall into a deep sleep, the muscles in the tongue, throat and roof of the mouth relax. This muscle relaxation causes the throat tissues to sag. This narrows the airway and creates the sound of snoring. If this were the end of it, then we would be looking at treating the noise and giving the family peace at night.

SLEEP APNOEA

However, for some people, snoring is dangerous. It is reported that 4% of males and 2% of females suffer obstructive sleep apnoea (OSA).[194] This breathing disorder is characterised by the repeated collapse of the upper airway during sleep and cessation of breathing.

---

[188] "Snoring and Sleep Apnoea". Snoring health fact sheet from BUPA. http://hcd2.bupa.co.uk/fact_sheets/Mosby_factsheets/snoring.html
[189] Halstrom, Wayne, "Snoring: The Universal Language. Dentistry offers a solution", *Oral Health*, Nov 1994
[193] Chambers 20th Century Dictionary, 1983
[194] Johal, A & Battagel, J M, "Current principles in the management of obstructive sleep apnoea with mandibular advancement appliances", *British Dental Journal*. Vol. 190, No. 10, May 26th, 2001

Subjects complain of excessive daytime sleepiness, headaches and impaired cognitive ability. Their partners frequently complain of the disruptive snoring with associated restlessness and involuntary leg movements during sleep. OSA subjects are at risk from severe medical complications, including hypertension, coronary heart disease and stroke as a result of nocturnal hypoxaemia (deficiency of oxygenation of the blood) and hypercapnia.

FLATTENED FACE
It is thought that the cause of this condition is skeletal. A retro-positioned facial skeleton and soft tissues (in a backward, closed-up position) reduces the oro-pharyngeal dimensions and impairs the function of the muscles of the upper airway. Overweight, smoking and alcohol intake are considered contributory factors to snoring and should be reduced where possible.

LIFESTYLE CHOICES
There is a large body of evidence which links snoring and OSA to the development of hypertension and high blood pressure.[195] Several studies have shown an increased risk of hypertension and cardiovascular diseases in snorers. It is also common to expect the snorer as well as the OSA patient to exhibit obesity. Disturbed breathing patterns during sleep act to reduce energy levels, producing tendencies to poor lifestyle choices that invite excess weight.

CUT-THROAT TREATMENT OPTION
Treatment has been varied over the years. At one time, tracheotomy was recommended. Not popular and rather excessive, however it did bypass the problem. But then, who wants to have their throat cut to stop the snoring? I guess a few wives have contemplated this, but it was seen as an unacceptable option, reserved for only the most severe OSA cases.

RESPIRATOR DEVICE
The respirator-device known as *nasal continuous positive air pressure* is also used for this condition. The patient wears a mask

---

[195] Halstrom, Wayne, ibid.

which fits over the nose, forming an airtight seal. A hose connects to an air pump beside the bed. A continuous airflow holds the airway open and relieves the apnoea. This is uncomfortable to wear, causes drying of the facial skin, is itself noisy and results in a reduction of patient compliance - to say nothing of its appeal to the bed partner! It is estimated that between 60 and 70% of people stop using this treatment in the long term and this low compliance has led to the need for a comfortable alternative.

STICK OUT THAT JAW
The treatment of snoring and OSA falls under three categories: surgical, medical and dental. Dentistry has provided a conservative way of dealing with this problem. The use of mandibular advancement splints, dental appliances that bring the lower jaw forward, is being increasingly recognised. The rationale for the use of MAS is that they may act to increase the size of the pharyngeal airway or otherwise reduce its collapsibility.

Another widely accepted theory on snoring believes that the problem lies in the tongue. As the person falls asleep, the tongue has a tendency to drop back and close up the airway, partially occluding the breathing which will result in snoring. Complete obliteration of the airway causes temporary periods of asphyxia or apnoea. Irrespective of the causative factors, bringing the lower jaw forward appears to relieve the problem for many suffering snorers.

AT THE FOREFRONT OF TREATMENT OPTIONS
At a research level, this treatment still appears quite new. Research often lags way behind what we are already doing in practice. Pulling the lower jaw forward for the relief of temporo-mandibular joint disorders has been recommended by Harold Gelb for years. Another dentist who had worked extensively in the field of jaw problems was Bill Farrar. While Gelb designed a piece of plastic for the lower jaw that encouraged the lower jaw forward as the teeth came together, Farrar opted for an upper appliance. This plastic worn over the upper teeth has a tag that hangs downwards from behind the upper front teeth and sits behind the lower front teeth when the jaws are opposed. The tag is long enough to prevent the lower jaw slipping backwards during sleep. The jaw is held forward on the lower teeth, the tongue is kept forward and the

palate remains activated and therefore doesn't appear to have the slackness with occlusion of the airway that is described above.

THANKS TO BILL FARRAR
I found the Farrar appliance beneficial in the reduction of snoring quite by chance. I had been in the practice of prescribing this appliance in combination with a daytime Gelb appliance. Patients would report that since wearing the upper appliance, snoring had decreased. Researchers would classify these observations as anecdotal, for lack of official research. For those of us in practice, this is on-the-job research, based on the powers of observation and recurrent confirmation by patients of the positive effects the appliance had on snoring.

According to Raphaelson and Alpher, dental appliance therapy may best be reserved for patients with primary snoring or with very mild sleep apnoea.[196] However, some patients with more severe problems have been helped with splints, when other treatments have failed.

OFF-THE-SHELF OR CUSTOM MADE?
With every problem, there is a man out there trying to solve it and make a living too. Manufacturers are attempting to replace the laboratory technician with 'one size fits all' appliances. This removes the necessity for dental impressions. While this can be unpleasant for some, it results in a custom-built appliance that fits only you. With mouths of very different shapes and sizes, this approach has its definite advantages.

TECHNOLOGY OR MARKETING?
The company information on 'off-the-shelf' appliances reads well and is certainly persuasive. Personally, I have found these appliances bulky and difficult for the person to wear. I fitted one on the doctor described earlier, but he found it difficult. I replaced it with a Farrar appliance and the patient is now comfortable with the smaller size, custom-built variety.

---

[196] Raphaelson, M, Alpher, E J, Bakker, K and Perlstrom, J "Oral Appliance Therapy for Obstructive Sleep Apnoea Syndrome: Progressive Mandibular Advancement During Polysomnography", *Journal of Cranio-Mandibular Practice*, 1998

A MATTER OF EXPERIENCE

Not all dentists are used to using splints, so 'off-the-shelf' devices are a great advantage for them. These come with good instructions and allow the novice to use the product satisfactorily. Not everything works for everyone. Indeed, one paper lists 5 categories of snoring, showing that appliances may only work for some grades:

- *Simple palatal level snoring*
- *Single level palatal obstruction.*
- *Palatal level obstruction with intermittent oropharyngeal involvement.*
- *Sustained multi-segment involvement.*
- *Tongue-base level obstruction.* [197]

AVOID SURGERY

According to this research, patients with grade 5 respond best to MAS therapy. Patients with grade 4 and 3 may also respond well, while grades one and two may be more ideal for surgery. I stand in favour of a non-invasive approach and will always attempt treatment rather than surgery. Surgery must be a last resort. Although oral appliances are effective in some patients with obstructive sleep apnoea, they are not universally effective.[198]

A novel anterior mandibular positioner (AMP) has been developed with an adjustable hinge that allows progressive advancement of the mandible. It was compared for efficacy, side-effects, patient compliance and preference between AMP and nasal continuous airway positive airway pressure (nCPAP) in patients with symptomatic mild to moderate OSA. Of these patients, one dropped out, three wouldn't cross over from one treatment to the other and only twenty people completed the trial. Of these twenty, eleven of them were treatment successes for the AMP, one couldn't cope and eight were failures. Fourteen of the twenty patients who used the nCPAP were treatment successes, six couldn't cope and

---

[197] Johal, A & Battagel, J, ibid.

[198] Ferguson, K, Takashi O, Lowe, A et al. "A short-term controlled trial of an adjustable oral appliance for the treatment of mild to moderate obstructive sleep apnoea", *Thorax*, 1997, 52: 362-368

there were no treatment failures. There was greater satisfaction with the AMP but no difference in side-effects or compliance.

DENTAL APPLIANCES GET THE THUMBS-UP

It was concluded that the AMP was effective in treating some patients with mild to moderate OSA and is associated with greater patient satisfaction than nCPAP.

In the dental office, this is another area of treatment that can be offered by your dentist. It is relatively easy to perform and with a reasonable chance of success, is certainly worth considering. While it may not always work, I recommend to my patients who do wear splints, that they use them for a minimum of six months. When first used, the appliance often finds its way to the bottom of the bed, under the pillow or on the floor. People actually take them out in their sleep. Perseverance is required and after about three weeks a good level of compliance can be achieved.

PEACE AT LAST

I believe that the benefits of mandibular advancement, good sleep, more energy and less risk of cardiovascular problems outweigh the disadvantages of a few sleepless nights and a reduction in the bank balance. For the partner and the relationship, this method of treatment must be seen as a positive step forward, giving peace at last!

We Are What We Absorb!

"Food is one of man's most immediate points of contact with nature. Man's sustenance must be suited to the laws that govern his body. Our ability to adapt cannot stretch beyond narrow limits." [199]

During the second half of the 19th century, French physiologist Claude Bernard pointed out that the internal environment of a living organism must remain fairly constant, despite changes in the external environment.

Some fifty years later the distinguished physiologist, Walter B Cannon suggested that this be called homeostasis: *"The ability of the body to maintain its internal environment despite external influences."* [200]

THE ROMANS

The Romans developed sophisticated flour-milling technology, producing 'fine flour' that was almost up to modern standards. Their flour had a creamier look, as the milling technique ground the wheat germ and much of the bran so finely that they could not be separated. It is interesting to note that their wrestlers ate only the coarse, wheaten bread in order to preserve the strength of their limbs. It had been realised that the milling and sieving process in some way denatured the food, making it less nutritious. But white is white, and the desire for the look appears to have outweighed the need for good nutrition.

FALL OF THE ROMAN EMPIRE

This decline in nutrition during the Roman era brought an increase in dental caries, assuming that there is a correlation between consumption of refined food and the incidence of tooth decay.[201] With the decline of the Roman Empire, there came a decline in this sophisticated process and a decline in caries rate

---

[199] Giedon S, *Mechanisation Takes Command,* Oxford Univ. Press, 1948
[200] Selye, Hans, *Stress without Distress*, ibid.
[201] Hall, Ross Hume, *Food for Nought*, Harper & Row, 1984

until about 1000 AD, when caries levels started to climb again to the levels that we see today.

By 1890, we had the automated flour mills of today. We had managed to remove the bran and germ leaving the starchy endosperm in the form of white, highly refined flour. The standard diet of the 19th century British working classes became white bread, jam and tea.[202] The deterioration in the physical condition and general health of the British masses became particularly noticeable by 1899. That this food had become empty is of no doubt. The people were malnourished due to the loss of the very life of the food that they were eating. The good had been removed, leaving something that was good to look at, marketable, enjoyed by the public but of little nutritional value.

EMPTY FOODS
Having realised that the flour is empty, there has been an effort to fortify this food, enriching it with thiamine, riboflavin, niacin, iron, and sometimes calcium. It would appear that at great cost we strip the goodness out of the grain and then at a further cost we replace it!

A report to the US Select Committee on Nutrition and Human Needs in February 1977 stated:

"Presently, we are a nation of sugarholics eating hollow, overcooked, government-inspected canned and packaged foods with 20-80% of the nutrition destroyed in processing. Breakfast cereals are a good example. Tests show that the paper boxes often contain more nutrition than all of the cereal contents. The nutrients in the wood pulp are still present while the overly processed cereals are quite devoid of nutritional value." [203]

SMART IS NOT ALWAYS SO SMART!
It is truly amazing that Dr Weston Price found tribes around the world with very little disease, no tooth decay, great physiques

---

[202] Burnett J, *Plenty and Want; A Social History of Diet in England from 1815 to the Present Day*, England, Penguin Books, 1968
[203] Fonder, Aelred, The Dental Physician, ibid.

and needing no prisons. Yet they lived on a so-called 'primitive' diet. Even more amazing is the fact that this diet was different, depending upon where they lived. They ate what they could find. They knew what to eat and they lived healthy lives. We 'got smart', found agriculture, refinement, preservatives and disease.

Not satisfied with causing our own demise, we then traded with these tribesmen so that they too could enjoy the same diseases and degeneration prevalent in Western society today - technology founded on mechanistic laws that clashed head on with the utterly diverse laws of the natural world. [204]

WHO ARE THE PRIMITIVE ONES?

The so-called 'primitive' races have been more efficient than modernised groups in the matter of preventing degenerative processes, physical, mental and moral, because they have been more efficient in complying with nature's laws. Dr Price conclusively proved this through his research of groups such as the Peruvian Incas, of whom he said:

"It is probable that few, if any of the ancient or modern cultures of the world have ever attained a more highly perfected organisation of society."[205]

The ruling Inca absolutely practised what he preached.

The Maori of New Zealand developed callisthenics and systematic physical exercise to a high degree. In his research of 250 skulls, Price found carious teeth in only two of them.

NO DENTIST, NO PHYSICIAN

The Australian Torres Strait Islanders were a happy, contented people who lived on seafood and tropical plants. Price studied Africans, Polynesians, Aborigines, Eskimaux and the Swiss from the Loetschental Valley. This last group had no dentist and no physician because they had no need for them. Their diet contained

---

[204] Hall, Ross Hume, ibid.
[205] Fonder, Aelred, ibid.

a high dairy content. Examination of their produce found it to be high in vitamins.

For these people it would appear that raw dairy produce was part of their staple diet and that they had the ability to metabolise it. Generally this does not seem to be the case with processed and denatured milk products today. In *Health Wars*, Phillip Day exposes the dangers of modern-day milk-consumption.[206]

All these people had one thing in common. While they ate a variety of foods, these foods were rich in nutrition. It was only when we introduced them to low-nutrition foods that they became susceptible to the same diseases as Western man.

PHYSICAL DEGENERATION
With the adoption of our white bread and sugar, the nutritional elements were no longer present to build sturdy bodies. The face became narrow, teeth were crowded, decay became a problem for the first time. The younger children were smaller. From being virtually non-existent, tuberculosis and arthritis rapidly became a problem. The narrowing of the pelvis, causing delayed births, also created many health problems for the mother and especially for the infant.[207]

What can we learn from these people? Back in the 1930's Weston Price stated:

"We have known for 40 years and more that the cause of physical degeneration is largely nutritional. May God help us if it takes another 40 years for our health professionals, the Food and Drug Administration, and our political and administrative office-holders to accept these facts." [208]

With cancer now striking approximately one in three and heart disease the leading killer within most industrialised societies today, we certainly need help.

---

[206] Day, Phillip, *Health Wars*, ibid.
[207] Price, Weston A, *Nutrition and Physical Degeneration*, ibid.
[208] Price, Weston A, ibid.

Dr Price found that, irrespective of the type of primitive diet, the latter's content was highly nutritious in contrast to the diet most Westerners consume today. Price's prediction that we would suffer increasing ill-health has tragically become a stark reality. What we can learn from these people is that we need to take action <u>immediately</u> and adopt a highly nutritious diet to give our bodies the raw materials they require to maintain and promote health. As Phillip Day sternly states: "If we don't do this, then suffer what we must suffer."

TOXINS, ALLERGENS, CARCINOGENS

There is another sinister player in the game. The foods that we eat contain toxins that are allergenic and carcinogenic. In his book *The Safe Shopper's Bible*, Dr Samuel Epstein points to two reports on pesticides in infants' and children's foods. These reports, prepared by the National Academy of Sciences and a Washington-based environmental working group, concluded that infants and children are at high risk from future cancers because of their exposure to carcinogenic pesticides. Dr. Epstein goes on to say that: *"Organically grown food is better, has more nutritional value and is low on toxins."* [209] However, as many of us already know, organic food is also expensive and often difficult to obtain.

ATHLETES

In her excellent book, *Strategies of the Champions*, Vicki Peterson highlights the diet of the Russian athletes.[210] She maintains that they are still way ahead of the West with their nutritional program. Yet it would appear that they have reinvented the wheel by turning back to the constituents of the less refined diet.

Their bread always contains the whole grain with black rye bread top of the list. The strengthening cereals start with millet and buckwheat, rye, oats and wheat. Cows' milk is fermented and mixed with the milk of ewes and goats.

---

[209] Steinman & Epstein, *Safe Shopper's Bible*, ibid.
[210] Peterson, Vicki, *Strategies of the Champions*, Sun Australia, 1991

Now, the idea of using milk may be confusing for those readers who picked up on the Casino milk affair mentioned earlier. However, the milk that we are talking about today is a far cry from the dairy produce of the Swiss people of the Loetsachental Valley. According to Weston Price, their dairy foods had a much higher mineral and vitamin content than commercial dairy products in America and Europe, and also had not been processed, skimmed, irradiated, pasteurised or otherwise denatured.[211]

The Russian athletes also used the omega 3 and 6 essential fatty acids, balanced their carbohydrate/protein ratio, ate raw vegetables which enhanced their immune system and used medicinal plants with pharmacologically active constituents. These foods enabled them to eat their way to health and success.

GONE TOO FAR

If it were practical, perhaps we would all return to the diet peculiar to our own country. It would appear though that technology and economics have gone too far for this to be a viable option. But we can buy organic or at least press for organic change and we can use nutritional supplementation to augment our empty foods. To this we can add antioxidants and herbal mixtures to protect the systems of the body. Taking in these nutrients is no more or less than we would have been doing naturally a few hundred years ago, were these foods available to us today in their whole, natural and unadulterated/unrefined state.

Athletes have realised the need to supplement the building blocks of the body. If you want to have a great immune system with cells that do what you want them to do, then you need to build good cells. Supplementation is like building a brick house. You can have all the cement in the world but without the bricks you don't have the house. So what is the body made of? [212]

Oxygen
Carbon
Hydrogen

---

[211] Fonder, Aelred, *The Dental Physician*, ibid.
[212] Hall, Ross Hume, *Food For Nought*, ibid.

Nitrogen
Calcium
Phosphorus
Potassium
Sulphur
Sodium
Chloride
Magnesium
Iron
Manganese
Copper
Iodine
Cobalt
Fluorine
Zinc
Chromium
Molybdenum
Selenium

WHAT DO WE NEED?

Vitamin A: Strengthens bones and helps in the formation and maintenance of the teeth and gums. How often have I heard patients say, *"My teeth are okay but my gums are falling out!"* or *"There was nothing wrong with my teeth but they took them all out because they were loose."* If you want to keep your teeth, you've got to have good bone. If you want good bone then nutrition is the cornerstone.

The B Vitamins: As a complex include B1 (thiamin), B2 (riboflavin), B3 (niacin), B5 (pantothenic acid) B6 (pyridoxine) and B12 (cyanocobalamin). These help the nervous system, reduce oral pain and regenerate blood cells.

Vitamin B17/Laetrile: Important as part of the cancer regimen.[213] Can be obtained through supplementation or through consumption of the nitriloside food group. Cultures whose diet is well mineralised and rich in nitrilosides do not contract cancer, as long as they are living in toxin-free environments. Oral cancers are

---

[213] Day, Phillip, *Cancer, Why We're Still Dying to Know The Truth*, ibid.

a difficult cancer to treat by the admission of the Western medical fraternity. In *'Cancer: Why We're Still Dying to Know the Truth'*, Phillip Day gives real hope and dispels the fears behind cancer and aggressive oral cancers.

Vitamin C: Important for the growth and repair of tissue cells, blood vessels, bones and teeth. Jacques Cartier witnessed the dramatic effects of sudden Vitamin C depletion in his crew, when his ship was marooned in the St Lawrence River in 1535.[214] Cartier's own words depict the state of the mouths of his shipmates as this deficiency took hold:

"Their mouths became stinking, their gums so rotten, that all the flesh did fall off, even the roots of the teeth which did almost all fall out."

Cartier was witnessing the breakdown of the elastin and collagen fibres that make up the gingival and arterial tissues of the mouth. Except for those whose sickly conditions were too far advanced, Cartier saw a rapid reversal of this disease with the administration of Vitamin C by means of a beverage containing maritime pine bark, given to him by the Indians of the region.

The post operative use of Vitamin C to heal wounds, to prevent bleeding or receding gums and to reduce gingival inflammation is recommended by New York dentist, Marc Lazare DDS. [215]

Vitamin D: maintains blood calcium levels by increasing dietary absorption of calcium and the reduction of calcium in the urine. It also helps in the utilisation of phosphorus. Deficiencies can lead to osteoporosis, soft bones and teeth (rickets), tooth decay and gum disease. Bone loss through periodontal disease has always been blamed on poor oral hygiene. As the nutrition story unfolds it becomes evident that these nutrients are essential if we are to keep our teeth and not lose them due to lack of bony support.

---

[214] Day, Phillip, *Health Wars*, ibid.
[215] Lazare, Marc,
www.ebody.com/cosmetic_dentistry/articles/199911/articles83.html

Vitamins are vitally important as part of the oral care program. They play an important part in the prevention of periodontal disease and in preventing the breakdown of gingival tissue. They help combat bleeding, swollen gums, tooth mobility, decay and halitosis. They help in the fight against oral infections and aid in the immune response. It must be said though that without the minerals they cannot be absorbed or utilised. It used to be that we obtained these minerals from the soils, but with intensive farming and poor crop rotation, this is no longer the case.

Macrominerals: Essential for the body. Minerals are classified as macrominerals if the recommended dietary allowance exceeds 100mg per day.

Calcium
Phosphorus
Potassium
Sulphur
Sodium
Chlorine
Magnesium

Microminerals: Trace minerals are those needed in quantities of less than 100mg per day. Although taken in smaller amounts, sometimes only a few micrograms a day, they are still essential to the body.

Iron
Manganese
Copper
Iodine
Cobalt
Fluorine
Zinc
Chromium
Molybdenum
Selenium
Nickel
Tin
Vanadium

HOW TO CHOOSE GOOD SUPPLEMENTS -
A BIT OF THIS, A BIT OF THAT?

Research shows that these elements and more are required to make good cells. Yet when asked about their supplementation, many of my patients answer, *"A bit of this and a bit of that."*

The difficulty can be knowing what to take. You walk into the local health food store intent on buying the best. Maybe it's your first time. You open the door, look in, and before your eyes is a plethora of colourful bottles of all shapes and sizes, promising everything you ever wanted. Eternal youth in a bottle, the skin of a sixteen-year-old when you're seventy, pills for your sagging bits, blood-vessel cleaners, waterworks modifiers, purges, potions and plenty of brain food.

In reality, if you approach the problem with logic, the answer is very simple: you need a good daily nutritional baseline in supplements, and then clean water, clean food, clean air and a clean environment.

NUTRITIONAL BASELINE -
VITAMIN AND MINERAL INTAKES

There are a number of companies today who do a single liquid ionised mineral and vitamin supplement which contains a whole host of these essential nutrients. Remember, minerals are required for vitamins to do their work. The huge rise in incidences of cancer and other degenerative diseases are primarily due to the depleted vitamin/mineral content in today's Western diet, coupled with environmental/chemical toxin factors.

The key nutritional ingredients invariably missing for cancer, for instance, are Vitamins B17, C, A, E and the trace mineral selenium. A recent US study showed an overall drop of 50% in cancer deaths and a fall of 37% in new cancer cases, especially lung, bowel and prostate – among 1,300 volunteers taking supplements for four years.[216] Mineral supplementation is most effective in the ionised 'liquid suspension' colloidal form, where an exceptionally

---

[216] *Daily Mail*, 28th July 1999, p. 31

high assimilation of the nutrients by the body is expected, as against other forms of minerals, such as the metallic variety. Our bodies use minerals as raw material. These cannot be manufactured by the body and so have to be present in the food and liquids we ingest. Sadly, as mentioned previously, our food chain is severely depleted of minerals, due to overfarming, fertilising effects and pesticide use. This has resulted in over 150 nutritional deficiency diseases that are now striking our societies with increasing intensity.[217]

To combat this very real threat, mineral and vitamin supplementation, far from being a quaint health fad, <u>is essential for everyone</u> and can literally make the difference between life or death, especially for those with cancer.

ANTIOXIDANTS/VITAMIN C
Scientists tell us that vitamins A, C, and E, as well as beta carotene and other antioxidant bioflavonoids, are vitally important to good health. But there are antioxidant formulae around now that have many more times the power of Vitamin C and Vitamin E. Current theory holds that oxidation elements, or free radicals as they are sometimes known, damage healthy cells when they rob electrons to render themselves stable. Ongoing free-radical activity comes about when we live in a polluted environment – even our own homes! Antioxidants such as Vitamin C neutralise the damage caused by free radicals. More powerful antioxidant material on the market today however, such as the oligomeric proanthocyanidins (OPC's) (see below), is very good news for all who care about their health. Every individual should ensure a good intake of antioxidants, to combat the destructive effects of our modern-day environments. Adequate intakes of antioxidants simply cannot be achieved through the regular Western diet.

Scurvy is a nutrition deficiency disease. It presents with widespread clinical pathological conditions of the supporting tissues of blood vessels, bones and teeth. There is also capillary fragility, which leads to bleeding and bruising. This is now a rare phenomenon, but chronic deficiency states of ascorbic acid are

---

[217] Day, Phillip, *Health Wars*, ibid.

more common than yesterday's scurvy and have been linked to chronic heart disease, the industrialised nations' number one disease killer.[218] A Vitamin C imbalance may also be manifested by impaired wound-healing and chronic gingivitis with a tendency to haematoma formation.

The gingivitis is an early manifestation. As the deficiency becomes more acute, the gums become grossly inflamed and bleed on slight pressure. At this point, the gums are highly susceptible to secondary infection. Calculus, poor oral hygiene and a poor bite aggravate this condition. Studies have shown that sub-clinical ascorbic acid deficiency increases the risk of periodontal disease.

The understanding that gum disease may be more than just poor oral hygiene must alert us to the need for vitamin supplementation in people with chronic gum problems. Vitamin C has been shown to be effective in treating scurvy and the protective effect can be increased manifold by the oligomeric proanthocyanidins (OPC's).

JACK MASQUELIER
Grape seed and pine bark extracts are a specific group of bio-flavinols and co-factors of Vitamin C, commonly known as OPC's or oligomeric proanthocyanidins. These were discovered and isolated by French scientist Jack Masquelier, who claims them to be 20 times more powerful than Vitamin C and 50 times more than Vitamin E. [219]

Dr Linus Pauling, often known as the 'Father of Vitamin C' and twice awarded the Nobel Prize, declared that large intakes of up to 10g of the vitamin each day aids anti-cancer activity within the body for cancer sufferers. Pauling was largely derided for making these declarations (yet he lived to be 94!), but today, large doses of Vitamin C are used by many practitioners for cancer patients in nutritional therapy, who believe Pauling was right and that the

---

[218] Rose, Louise F & Kaye, Donald, *Internal Medicine for Dentists*, The CV Mosby Company, 1990. For the heart disease connection, please see Day, Phillip, *Health Wars*, ibid.
[219] "Protecting the Cardiovascular System against Heart Disease and Stroke with Masquelier" http://www.pychealth.com/stroke.html

popular nutrient is indispensable to the body in its fight to regain health from cancer.

Several studies have suggested that Vitamin C may reduce levels of lead in the blood. Epidemiological studies have shown that people with elevated blood serum levels of Vitamin C had lower levels of blood toxicity. An examination of the data from the Third National Health and Nutrition Examination Survey, enrolling 4,213 youths aged 6 to 16 years and 15,365 adults 17 years and older from 1988 to 1994, found a correlation between low serum ascorbic acid levels and elevated blood lead levels. The authors conclude that high ascorbic acid intake may reduce blood lead levels.[220]

An analysis of the Normative Aging Study, which enrolled 747 men aged 49 to 93 years from 1991 to 1995, found that lower dietary intake of Vitamin C may increase lead levels in the blood.[221] A study of 349 African American women enrolled in the project Nutrition, Other Factors, and the Outcome of Pregnancy found that vitamin-mineral supplementation resulted in increased serum levels of ascorbic acid and decreased serum levels of lead. The authors concluded that maternal use of a vitamin supplement with ascorbic acid and Vitamin E might offer protection from lead contamination of the foetus during pregnancy.[222]

Because smoking lowers levels of ascorbic acid in the body, researchers theorised that Vitamin C supplementation may affect blood lead levels in smokers. A clinical study was performed on 75 adult men 20 to 30 years of age who smoked at least one pack of cigarettes per day, but had no clinical signs of ascorbic acid deficiency or lead toxicity. Subjects were randomly assigned to daily supplementation with placebo, 200 mg of ascorbic acid, or 1000 mg of ascorbic acid. After one week of supplementation, there was

[220] Simon J A, Hudes E S, "Relationship of Ascorbic Acid to Blood Lead Levels." *JAMA.* 1999;281:2289-2293.

[221] Cheng Y, Willett W C, Schwartz J, Sparrow D, Weiss S, Hu H, "Relation of nutrition to bone lead and blood lead levels in middle-aged to elderly men. The Normative Aging Study." *Am. J. Epidemiol.* 1998 Jun 15;147(12):1162-1174.

[222] West W L, Knight E M, Edwards C H, et al, "Maternal low level lead and pregnancy outcomes." *J. Nutr.* 1994 Jun;124(6 Suppl):981S-986S.

an 81% decrease in blood-lead levels in the group taking 1000 mg of ascorbic acid daily.[223]

IMPLEMENTING CHANGES –
CONVERTING YOUR BATHROOM

As many of the harmful ingredients we examined earlier can be found in the average bathroom, clear these out in one fell swoop and replace with safe and environmentally friendly alternatives (see *Contacts!* for advice on where to obtain these). At the moment, many of us are brushing our teeth with rat poison, washing our hair out with cheap engine degreasants, putting liquid paraffin on our babies in the form of baby oil, firing aluminium into the lymph nodes under our arms and using constituents of brake fluid and antifreeze in our make-up and personal care formulae. Does this make sense?

IMPLEMENTING CHANGES –
IMPORTANCE OF DIET

Again, a great, wholesome, organic diet cannot be stressed enough. Changes in diet are essential to avoid contracting a deficiency disease. As we have seen, the main culprit is the good old Western diet, heavy in meats, sugars, fats and chemicals. Removal of all potentially contaminated meats (replacing with a small element of organic meat), as well as removal of toxic foodstuffs such as additives, caffeine, refined sugars and chocolate represents a major start. Weight loss and a return of energy are almost immediate, and with these benefits comes a regular method of detoxifying the body as part of your future lifestyle.

Rapid detoxification can be achieved simply by eating more fruit in the morning between when you awaken and noon. Fruits such as pineapple, grapes (eat the seeds!), plums and oranges are among many that are ideal for this purpose and contain a vast array of nutrients, whose effectiveness and modality are only now beginning to be properly understood. If you are used to bulk in the mornings with the traditional breakfasts, eat more fruit and then

---

[223] Dawson EB, Evans DR, Harris WA, Teter MC, McGanity WJ "The effect of ascorbic acid supplementation on the blood lead levels of smokers." *J. Am. Coll. Nutr.* 1999 Apr;18(2):166-170.

wait for your raised blood sugars to remove your feelings of hunger. For concrete advice on these highly effective dietary regimens, and what to do if you are diabetic, please obtain a copy of Phillip Day's *Health Wars*, which gets into detail on diet detoxification measures to get you lean, trim, in the peak of health, and perhaps even more important – educated.[224]

Food is absolutely the most potent drug we put into our body and it is by far the most abused. If you want to find the root causes for all major diseases we are suffering from today, take a look at your supermarket cart next time you are lining up at the check-out. How much of it is WHOLE FOOD, UNPROCESSED, UNCONTAMINATED AND UNADULTERATED?

EXERCISE IN MODERATION

Research shows that those with a sedentary lifestyle are more prone to cancer and heart problems. A moderate exercise program will assist in cleansing the body and getting all the pieces of the body toned and in proper working order. Simply MOVE! Walking, a non-threatening hour in the gym twice or three times a week or cycling are ideal and immensely enjoyable once you get on the pro-active program. If you sit still all day long, you might as well not breathe! Life is about healthy action. Celebrate your life by looking, moving and feeling the way your body was designed to be.

---

[224] Day, Phillip, *Health Wars*, ibid.

Dentistry Reviewed

There are some topics that may have warranted a chapter in themselves, but I am including them in a Frequently Asked Question (FAQ) section, in the hope that they will spur you on to ask your dentist. I am aware that the system of dentistry is different around the world. For example, the National Health system in the UK is different from private practice. The materials and criteria for their use in the NHS are decided at government level. Under private contract, this can be decided between the dentist and patient.

PRIVATE DENTISTRY

For the sake of this discussion and the questions that follow, I have decided to look at private dentistry rather than the British NHS. Having worked both in Australia and the UK, I am aware that the ideology behind the NHS makes it a great system for those who cannot afford anything else. This is not to say that the treatment is poor, for it is not and there are many conscientious dentists working within the health service doing excellent work using the materials at their disposal. The use of low-grade crowns, filling materials and lack of time is the economic reality of an expensive system attempting to service a huge population. Under NHS contract, there are services that cannot, for obvious reasons of cost, be provided. The use of white fillings and white/porcelain crowns at the back of the mouth is not allowed under the NHS and some orthodontic treatments are not financially viable for the practitioner.

BATTLE-ZONE DENTISTRY

Having said that, what a great service we do provide with an emergency system manned by local dentists who attend local hospitals nightly to see and treat any dental emergency that comes through the door and at a cost no more expensive than any other item under the NHS service. This alone enables many people who are terrified of the dentist to attend as a last resort, knowing they will be helped. In some countries, a great deal of suffering goes on amongst the people who can't afford to pay. In the UK, if you can't afford it, you still get a level of treatment that means that you are out of pain. I like this. It is truly what dentistry and medicine should be all about.

I CAN'T WORK WITH MY
HANDS TIED BEHIND MY BACK!

The private system allows you, the end user, to get what you want. A treatment plan is formulated and agreed upon between you and your practitioner and work is commenced.

I favour this system as it allows me to work with my patients without compromise. I can use the latest materials such as posterior composite white fillings, white inlays and white porcelain or bonded crowns. I can embark on full TMJ/myofascial work and know that the fee structure is favourable to both parties. Basically, it's great to work without my hands tied behind my back.

I was recently reading of an American dentist who thought that he had made a major breakthrough. He could prepare a tooth for a crown in record time and charge a fortune for getting through the work rapidly and causing the patient the least amount of pain, inconvenience or time in the surgery. As dentists under NHS contract, we've been doing this for years!

The only difference is that he gets paid maybe £500 for his crown and under the NHS we get about £70. Why? Unfortunately, the government has decided what a crown should cost; we realised that if we did them quickly we would earn more per hour than if they were done slowly. In reply to this, our peers realised that our hourly rate had gone up so they dropped the price of the crown! Now we have to do them quickly to make any money at all.

That's fine if you can work fast and maintain a good standard. The slower dentists are financially penalised for this, while those with a system and the manual dexterity to go with it keep raking in the money. So, it's not all sweet under the NHS/Private Healthcare System. At least under private contract (as in the rest of the business world) you can decide what you are worth, what you want, what works between both parties, and enter into an agreement.

And now on to the Frequently Asked Questions section. These are some of the questions that routinely come up either in the surgery, over a meal or down at the pub. The list is not exhaustive but then, next time you see your dentist in a coffee shop, wine bar or bump into him or her in the supermarket, you can ask your own burning questions and see what answers they come up with.

Frequently Asked Questions

Q. *What dangers are there in submitting to dental X-rays?*

A. It depends on the regularity and why they are being taken. There is a great deal spoken about X-rays being linked to carcinogenicity and tissue damage. On 29th June 1981, before the National Centre for Health Care Technology Assessment Forum, Dr Lauriston S Taylor, Honorary President of the NCRP, made the following comments:

"The public tends to believe there is a much greater risk of harm from radiology than actually exists. The dose of radiation normally used in dental radiology is so low as to pose little if any risk. Nevertheless, because any exposure to radiation might possibly cause harm, X-rays should be used only when the patient is expected to benefit." [225]

X-rays are an important aid to treatment. They should be used with discretion and only when required. It is not always easy to see decay between teeth or under crowns, fillings and inlays. It is better to be able to treat the tooth before the decay has reached the nerve, than deal with the possibility of a root canal or extraction.

X-rays are of great value for surgical extractions and where buried roots are suspected. Quite often, a patient will present with toothache having worn dentures for years. X-rays reveal a buried root that is now a problem and requires removal. If you don't know how much is there, it is easy to get it wrong!

Periodontal infections and bone levels can be assessed using X-ray. Root infections, abscesses, cyst, traumatic fractures of both teeth and jaws, solitary bone cysts or NICO lesions can often be identified with X-ray. TMJ pathology, orthodontic therapy, pain of unknown dental cause all obviate the need for X-ray.

---

[225] Rose, Louise F, ibid.

That having been said, there is a body of evidence that shows X-ray energy to be cumulative, which can in the long term prove dangerous, in the absence of the body's ability to detoxify. So my caveat is this. Have X-rays if they are absolutely required.

Q. *Can we treat without X-rays?*
A. Yes. We treat pregnant women without X-ray, when they are in pain, and do all that we can to relieve them. But knowing that the scatter is slight, exposure time small and the benefits valuable, my considered opinion is that we continue with them until technology comes up with something different. We are starting to use computer-generated images and the government is not keen on the use of old machines with high exposure rates.

One word of caution. X-rays are an obvious area for abuse through financial gain per X-ray. It is not unknown for a dentist to take them more often than is absolutely necessary! Extremes are not good either. Some dentists never take X-rays. You might then change dentists and all of a sudden you genuinely need ten fillings.

If you have no problems, no pain and nothing going on and never had a filling, it's difficult to justify more than one set of X-rays to establish a baseline. If you have rampant decay and need fillings every six months, then you will need closer observation. The majority fall somewhere in between and as a guideline, bite wing X-rays (premolar and molar region) may be taken every 18 months to 2 years and the OPG (the big one that goes around your head) every 4-5 years. I like this X-ray for looking at bone levels, tooth position and to give some idea of the state of the jaw joints.

It is sad to think that with ever increasing litigation and ambulance chasing by greedy lawyers, X-rays may well increase in number.

Q. *Should I give my children fluoride tablets?*

A. See the section on fluoride. The use of fluoride must be one of personal choice. Based on the evidence, I cannot recommend fluoride for my patients.

According to a report by the Poison Information Centre in Vienna, accidental ingestion of sodium fluoride tablets for caries prophylaxis is a frequent event that does not usually present a serious risk.[226] It goes on to report the death of a 3 year-old boy after swallowing 200 tablets which equated to 16mg/kg body weight. Though the report indicates the cause of death as uncertain, the number of tablets swallowed was excessive. There is still a risk.

Fluoride has several mechanisms of toxicity.[227] Ingested fluoride acts on the intestinal mucosa. It can form hydrofluoric acid, which leads to gastric irritation. Once absorbed, fluoride binds to calcium ions and may lead to hypocalcaemia. It is cytotoxic to enzyme systems, causing increased salivation, vomiting and diarrhoea. Seizures may follow as a result of lowered magnesium and calcium. Severe fluoride toxicity will result in multi-organ failure.

We discussed the many ways that fluoride can enter the body. It is already difficult to regulate. Fluoride tablets can therefore be seen as just another way of increasing unnecessary fluoride load.

"Tooth decay is back—it's worse than ever—it's coming to a tooth near you!" said a dentist to a National Institutes of Health panel convened to evaluate tooth decay research, March 2001. [228] Most tooth decay research is poorly done, the panel concluded. Lack of fluoride doesn't cause decay, poor diet does!

"Whilst fluoride is proclaimed as a significant cavity reducer, there is little, if any, science to support that." says lawyer Paul Beeber, President, New York State Coalition Opposed to

---

[226] Eichler, H G, et al, "Accidental Ingestion of NaF Tablets by Children", *International Journal of Clinical Pharmacology, Therapy and Toxicology*, Vol. 20, No.7, 1982
[227] www.emedicine.com/emerg/topic181.htm
[228] NYS Coalition Opposed to Fluoridation, http://www.orgsites.com/ny/nyscof

Fluoridation. *"Furthermore, there's no evidence that lack of fluoride puts children at high risk for cavities."*[229]

Q. Do white fillings last as long as the mercury fillings?

A. I can only give a clinical view on this. I have seen amalgam fillings that have been in place for well over thirty years and there is no evidence of decay. Then I have seen white fillings that have been placed within a year to eighteen months and decay is present. However, do remember from the chapter on fillings that over 60% of all restorative work carried out under the NHS is to redo work that has already been done.

Historically, we know that amalgam fillings have been used for over 150 years. As a filling material it's great. Easy to use, strong once set and remains for years. White fillings in back teeth are a fairly recent event. When I qualified in 1977, we were not using posterior white fillings as there was doubt over strength and durability. These early fillings were chemically cured by mixing two products together, a base and a catalyst. Now the filling materials are light-cured and are highly sophisticated. The manufacturers assure us that they are wear-resistant and capable of withstanding the biting forces placed on back teeth.

On balance, one still has to admit that white fillings don't last as long as amalgams. It would appear however that they are also not as toxic as amalgams to the body. One could argue that if you have a known toxin in the body for a long period of time, this presents a problem for the immune system and may lead to sensitivity or allergy. The immuno-toxicologists show us that people who are sensitive to heavy metals are sensitive to amalgams also. If you wear metal earrings and suffer weepy ears as a result, you are almost certainly sensitive to heavy metals and shouldn't have amalgam fillings either.

BIO-COMPATABILITY

What you are looking for in a filling is the most bio-compatible material available. Many non-amalgam dentists choose the glass

---

[229] Beeber, Paul, ibid.

ionomer filling materials which appear the most bio-compatible. Others choose a mixture of glass ionomer/composite. These are the compomers. The drawback with these is that they also release fluoride. Composites are still popular. Whether in the future we find these toxic to the system remains to be seen. The use of laboratory-made composites as inlays is also an option. These are fillings made by the technician and then sent to the dentist for placing in the mouth.

The problem of filling choice and placement becomes increasingly more difficult. I have just received an e-mail on glass ionomers. According to The Department of Human Work Sciences in Sweden, this product is cytotoxic. It releases aluminium and fluoride at a cytotoxic level.[230] This poses a problem for the dentist attempting to place the most biocompatible non-toxic substance into the body.

I would qualify my answer in this way: if it were my wife or child, I would use composite inlays. Where possible, I would use all porcelain crowns such as 'inceram' or 'procera' and if the cavity only warranted a filling, I would use composite instead of amalgam.

Q. *Why are white fillings more expensive than amalgams*?
A. They take longer to place than amalgams. The material is great but not as easy to use, nor as forgiving.

Q. *Do I need antibiotics?*
A. Patients sometimes visit for emergency repairs before a foreign holiday. They request a prescription *'just in case',* in the belief that the level of dentistry skills abroad might well be lower or so expensive that if anything should go wrong, they could fall back on those 'magic bullets,' otherwise known as antibiotics.

---

[230] Lonnroth E C, Dahl J E, "Cytotoxicity of Dental Glass Ionomers Evaluated using Dimethylthiazol Diphenyltetrazolium and Neutral Red Tests", www.entrez-PubMed.org

STOP ANTIBIOTICS ON DEMAND

According to two endodontists, John W Harrison, DMD, MS, Professor of Endodontics, Baylor College of Dentistry, Dallas and Richard E Walton, DMD, MS, Professor of Endodontics, College of Dentistry, University of Iowa, Iowa City, *"We have to end the era of antibiotics on demand."* [231]

Drs Harrison and Walton say there is no scientific evidence that antibiotics ease toothache pain or swelling, nor that they contribute to speed-healing after root-canal procedures. But there is considerable evidence that they pose a risk to the patient and to the population as a whole. There is overwhelming evidence of the emerging problem of bacterial resistance to antibiotics.

JUSTIFICATION FOR ANTIBIOTIC USE

The guidelines for antibiotic use are facial swelling, swollen glands, fever and difficulty opening the mouth. Pain is not in this criteria, as set out by the American Association of Endodontists. They remind us that each time we use them, we are contributing to the development of resistant strains of bacteria.

ECHINACEA: A SAFE OPTION

It is rare for me to prescribe antibiotics. One safe alternative to take on holiday is Echinacea. I have found it to be useful for everything from coughs and colds to oral infections that don't require antibiotics. At the first sign of a cold or flu my staff and I reach for an Echinacea supplement with great results. Here's a good product to pack for your holidays!

Q. *Should I take calcium for my periodontal bone loss?*

A. Calcium is a macro-mineral, found in the skeleton, that gives bones their strength. Calcium is the most abundant element in the human body. It is required for proper muscle contraction, maintenance of a slight alkali pH in the blood, blood clotting and nerve maintenance. Low serum calcium can lead to muscle cramps and tetany (muscle spasms). Osteoporosis is caused in almost all

---

[231] American Association of Endodontists, 56th Annual Session, Atlanta, Georgia, USA, 23rd April 1999

cases by, you guessed it, an acidic body system (diet is the major culprit). One of the easiest ways to prevent osteoporosis is to maintain an alkalised internal environment so the body does not need to strip minerals from the bone structure to maintain its desired alkali.[232]

MAGNESIUM

Magnesium deficiency can lead to a drop in calcium levels. The relationship between magnesium and calcium is similar to that between sodium and potassium, and magnesium itself is directly involved in the regulation of potassium. The latter is mainly intra-cellular.

One of the difficulties with calcium is that as we get older, it is less readily absorbed. I do not routinely prescribe calcium for my patients but it is well worth considering as part of the overall nutritional program. A calcium lactate solution with Magnesium and Vitamin D is the best to use along with sunlight, in order to increase the absorption of the calcium.

Q. Can I get mouth cancer?

A. More than 2,500 new cases of oral cancer are diagnosed every year and about 1,400 people die from the disease.[233] Conventional treatment is not particularly successful, hence the 50% death rate. Smoking, excessive alcohol drinking and chewing tobacco all increase the risk of cancer. More common amongst men, these cancers are found on the side of the tongue, behind the back teeth and on the floor of the mouth. Your dentist will screen you for this at your check-up and, if suspicious, will refer you to an oral surgeon for further investigation. If you are worried, you should seek advice. Spend a few days going over Phillip Day's *Cancer: Why We're Still Dying to Know The Truth* for excellent anti-cancer strategies for the whole family.

---

[232] Day, Phillip, *Health Wars*, ibid.
[233] "High Death Rate in Oral Cancer", www.lineone.net/skynews/uk/story/1999

CARE FOR YOUR DENTIST
HE/SHE CARES FOR YOU

There are many questions about dentistry. Hopefully, your dentist and staff will be able to answer yours for you. Remember, that while receiving dental treatment may not be the most pleasurable experience in the world, the informed dentist really does want what is best for you. But there is a tremendous amount every member of the public can do to avoid needless pain and heartache within their own body and within the family. Make use of the information contained in this book and, most importantly, become fully educated on all things related to teeth.

Knowledge is Power, as they say, and this knowledge can be the power of a pain-free and enjoyable, fulfilling life, where the alternative used to be misery, pain and disease. Spread the word, spread the information in this book, and ENJOY YOUR LIFE!

And Finally...

"When great changes occur in history, when great principles are involved, as a rule the majority are wrong."[234]

In putting this book together, I have attempted to highlight the different areas of dentistry that could be responsible for making you sick. Selye's model has run as a constant theme throughout the book:

"Stress is the non-specific reaction of the body to any demand placed upon it."

Once we understand that it is what we do to ourselves and what is done to us that ultimately affects our lives, we can begin to gain control of our health and well-being.

In the quest for good health we need to address the issues covered in this book:

Great diet – Eat organically grown, pesticide-free, living whole foods, a high percentage of which should be eaten raw.

Great nutritional supplements - choose a company whose expertise is well known and whose products have a great track record of efficacy. Baseline nutrition should include a highly bio-available vitamin and mineral supplement. Some on the market also come with rare earths, amino acids, enzymes and other co-factors. An antioxidant supplement and other simple nutrients recommended in Phillip Day's *Health Wars* are also advised.

Good oral hygiene – Brush properly and regularly after meals, floss and use a safe, effective mouthwash.

Balancing of the bite

Replacement of missing teeth

Good dentistry

Safe products – Use toothpastes and mouthwashes without sodium fluoride, and change your other personal care products,

---

[234] Debs, Eugene V, speech at his trial, Cleveland, Ohio, 12th September, 1918

such as shampoo, conditioner, make-up, deodorants, etc. for the safe alternatives.

Eradication of toxins – Rid your food, water and environment of known toxin problems

Safety for the children – Ensure a safe, nutritious environment for your children and train them up in health habits that will last them a lifetime.

Drink plenty of clean, pure water (at least 2 litres/4 pints a day)

"Do you not know that your body is the temple of the Holy Spirit who is in you, whom you have from God, and you are not your own?

For you were bought at a price; therefore glorify God in your body and in your spirit, which are God's." **1 Corinthians: 19-20**.

Why Are The Nations Dying?

Degenerative diseases are taking hold of industrialised nations like never before. The following excerpted US Senate document warned of the health holocaust to come.

Senate Document No. 264, 1936
74th Congress, 2nd Session

"Our physical well-being is more directly dependent upon minerals we take into our systems than upon calories or vitamins, or upon precise proportions of starch, protein or carbohydrates we consume... Do you know that most of us today are suffering from certain dangerous diet deficiencies which cannot be remedied until depleted soils from which our food comes are brought into proper mineral balance?

The alarming fact is that foods (fruits, vegetables and grains), now being raised on millions of acres of land that no longer contain enough of certain minerals, are starving us - no matter how much of them we eat. No man of today can eat enough fruits and vegetables to supply his system with the minerals he requires for perfect health because his stomach isn't big enough to hold them.

The truth is, our foods vary enormously in value, and some of them aren't worth eating as food... Our physical well-being is more directly dependent upon the minerals we take into our systems than upon calories or vitamins or upon the precise proportions of starch, protein or carbohydrates we consume.

This talk about minerals is novel and quite startling. In fact, a realization of the importance of minerals in food is so new that the text books on nutritional dietetics contain very little about it. Nevertheless, it is something that concerns all of us, and the further we delve into it the more startling it becomes.

You'd think, wouldn't you, that a carrot is a carrot - that one is about as good as another as far as nourishment is concerned? But it isn't; one carrot may look and taste like another and yet be lacking in the particular mineral element which our system requires and which carrots are supposed to contain.

Laboratory test prove that the fruits, the vegetables, the grains, the eggs, and even the milk and the meats of today are not what they were a few generations ago (which doubtless explains why our forefathers thrived on a selection of foods that would starve us!)

No man today can eat enough fruits and vegetables to supply his stomach with the mineral salts he requires for perfect health, because his stomach isn't big enough to hold them! And we are turning into big stomachs.

No longer does a balanced and fully nourishing diet consist merely of so many calories or certain vitamins or fixed proportion of starches, proteins and carbohydrates. We know that our diets must contain in addition something like a score of minerals salts.

It is bad news to learn from our leading authorities that 99% of the American people are deficient in these minerals [this was in 1936!], **and that a marked deficiency in any one of the more important minerals actually results in disease. Any upset of the balance, any considerable lack or one or another element, however microscopic the body requirement may be, and we sicken, suffer, shorten our lives.**

We know that vitamins are complex chemical substances which are indispensable to nutrition, and that each of them is of importance for normal function of some special structure in the body. Disorder and disease result from any vitamin deficiency. **It is not commonly realized, however, that vitamins control the body's appropriation of minerals, and in the absence of minerals they have no function to perform. Lacking vitamins, the system can make some use of minerals, but lacking minerals, vitamins are useless. Certainly our physical well-being is more directly dependent upon the minerals we take into our systems than upon calories of vitamins or upon the precise proportions of starch, protein of carbohydrates we consume.**

This discovery is one of the latest and most important contributions of science to the problem of human health."

The Vitamin C 'Scare'

by Steven Ransom
Credence Research

The following article is reprinted in full from Credence archives. Its findings prove most relevant to the debate on how Big Business, Big Pharma and Big Government are trying to monopolise all sectors of public health through scare tactics and false propaganda.

THEY SAY THAT VITAMIN C
CAN INCREASE THE RISK OF CANCER
Oh yes? And who's 'they'?

VITAMIN C CANCER FEAR - *High doses of Vitamin C could increase the risk of cancer, scientists warn today....*

So begins the 15th June 2001 UK Daily Mail front-page report, outlining the work of Dr Ian Blair, resident researcher at the University of Pennsylvania Pharmacology Unit. The Mail headline appears to be in direct conflict with Dr Blair's own statement: "Absolutely, for God's sake, don't say Vitamin C causes cancer." (Yahoo News, Thursday, 14th June 2001) But of course, The Mail and others have shamelessly done exactly that. To the less discerning reader, the story raises worrisome questions as to the wisdom of high-level Vitamin C supplementation. If these worldwide headlines have served any useful purpose at all, it has been to confirm the moral/intellectual void currently reigning in today's mass media 'news' departments.

CASTING ASPERSIONS

At a more fundamental level, why is Dr Blair conducting tests on the efficacy of Vitamin C at all? We are about to discover that certain parties have a very definite interest in casting aspersions upon Vitamin C. To our knowledge, the information you are about to read has not been included in any of the latest, and now worldwide **'Vitamin C Cancer Scare'** headlines generated by Dr Blair's findings.

A GOLDEN RULE

Dr Blair postulates that high consumption of Vitamin C (a most beneficial adjunct in non-toxic cancer recovery treatment) might actually cause human tissue degeneration, which in turn could lead to a heightened risk of contracting cancer. And it is here that we arrive at our first golden rule: when it comes to assessing the veracity of any scientific claim, we must <u>always</u> read between the lines – we must search for what the report <u>does not</u> say. We must especially be on the look-out for that hoary old chestnut, otherwise known as vested interests. A University of Manchester research methodology handbook contains the following valuable advice:

"Science and research must be studied in the context of all the interested parties involved. The questions centre on determining the relative weight of the various allies in the 'fact-creating' process - e.g. funding bodies, businesses, departments of state, professions and other scientists. In analysing scientific debates, <u>one should always ask what social, institutional, political and philosophical interests lie behind often apparently 'neutral' and 'technical' knowledge claims</u>." (University of Manchester Institute of Science & Technology (UMIST) research methodology course handout, 1994)

On the matter of the 'fact creation' process, renowned author John Le Carré recently stated:

"Big Pharma [the industry in general] *is engaged in the deliberate seduction of the medical profession, country by country, worldwide. It is spending a fortune on influencing, hiring and purchasing academic judgment to a point where, in a few years' time, if Big Pharma continues unchecked on its present happy path, unbought medical opinion will be hard to find."* (The Nation, New York, Interview with John Le Carré, 9th April 2001)

BOUGHT?

With the above in mind, let's put Dr Blair's University of Pennsylvania under the spotlight and see what encouragement Dr Blair might have had in taking his extraordinary and apparently misquoted position against Vitamin C. We must ask the following questions: what Big Pharma influences might there be supporting the University of Pennsylvania Cancer Center (UPCC) and its mother ship, the University of Pennsylvania Health Service? What is the relative weight of the funding bodies? If industry sponsorship is taking place, are UPHS personnel free to exercise unbiased, critical thinking? Or are there grounds to suspect that UPHS has been 'bought' - that somewhere along the line, vested interests have 'purchased academic judgment'? Before tackling the Vitamin C issue itself, the following UPHS general statistics are very revealing.

CERTAIN ALLIANCES
In May 2000, Dr Ian Blair's employers at UPCC received a $26 million, five-year Core Grant from the National Cancer Institute (NCI) - the largest and most influential conventional cancer treatment institution in the world. In fact, UPCC has been continuously funded by the NCI Core Grant mechanism since the grant was created by the National Cancer Act in the early 1970's. Currently, UPCC is awash with more than $100 million in cancer research funding: $37 million is from the National Cancer Institute; $43 million from closely affiliated organisations, such as the National Institutes of Health, the institution which actually funded Dr Blair's Vitamin C research; another $12 million from foundational support such as the American Cancer Society and the Leukaemia Society; and between $8 and $10 million from various pharmaceutical companies. Earlier, in June of 1999, UPCC received a $4.5 million gift from the William H. Gates Foundation to research conventional treatments for non-Hodgkin's lymphoma.

Aside from the Bill and Melinda Gates connection, OncoLink, the University of Pennsylvania Cancer Center, is sponsored very generously by the following corporations: Amgen, the world's largest independent biotechnology company; Aventis, Ortho Biotech, Inc., Varian, Inc., Janssen Pharmaceutica, AstraZeneca, Pharmacia Upjohn and Pfizer. These corporations are very big indeed, and their names represent no mean sponsorship committee.

MORE ALLIANCES
In March 2001, UPHS announced a strategic alliance with Siemens Medical Systems, Inc. Under the terms of the purchasing agreement, UPHS will make an initial discounted purchase of cardiology, radiology and radiation oncology equipment from Siemens, who will also service and maintain the biomedical equipment already in place at designated UPHS sites over the life of the agreement. In the year 2000, Siemens Medical Solutions, based in Iselin, New Jersey, reported new orders of $5.65 billion, sales of $5.44 billion and employs 27,000 worldwide.

"This is the kind of alliance that will be critical in our continuing financial recovery and to assure our position as a leading national health system," said Robert D. Martin, Ph.D., Chief Executive Officer of UPHS.

A good relationship with Siemens may well be critical to UPHS' financial recovery, but does this kind of dependent alliance foster the aforementioned necessary climate for critical thinking? What if there are privately held UPHS reservations over the Siemens equipment, methodology or ethos? Who will break rank first? Will anyone? What kind of commercially gagged framework are the UPHS staff now locked into with Siemens?

YET MORE CORPORATE ALLIANCES

On April 26, 2001, UPCC announced a business partnership with Integral PET Associates, the nation's leading operator of fixed-site Positron Emission Tomography (PET) cancer scanners. A patient receiving a PET scan today is injected with a radiopharmaceutical, such as flurodeoxyglucose (FDG), about 45 minutes before the scan, which takes about two hours. The radiopharmaceutical tracer emits signals which are then picked up by the PET scanner.

A computer reassembles the signals into recognisable images to determine if a cancer has spread, if a particular treatment is effective, or if a patient is disease-free. IPA will now be seeking to supply major hospitals throughout Pennsylvania with this very expensive equipment. Installing and operating a PET scanner typically costs around $1,600,000 in up-front capital costs, plus an additional $800,000 in yearly staff and operational costs.

A short visit to the UPHS website at www.med.upenn.edu will not only confirm all of the above information, but will also confirm that these alliances represent only a small percentage of the long-standing conventional 'friendships' UPHS has fostered with Big Pharma over the years. Given the strictly conventional source of sponsorship monies received at UPHS, what chance will the following statements have of being 'allowed' to feature on the UPHS cancer information page?

"If I contracted cancer, I would never go to a standard cancer treatment centre. Cancer victims who live far from such centres have a chance." **Professor Charles Mathe, French cancer specialist**

"...as a chemist trained to interpret data, it is incomprehensible to me that physicians can ignore the clear evidence that chemotherapy does much, much more harm than good." **Alan C Nixon, PhD, former president of the American Chemical Society**

"Doctors are too busy to dig into the statistics of cancer treatments, they assume that what they are taught at school or what is demonstrated in the pages of briefing journals is the best treatment. They cannot afford to suspect that these treatments are only the best for the pharmaceutical companies that influence their 'institutions of higher learning'." **Paul Winter, The Cancell Home Page.**

"To the cancer establishment, a cancer patient is a profit center. The actual clinical and scientific evidence does not support the claims of the cancer industry. Conventional cancer treatments are in place as the law of the land because they pay, not heal, the best. Decades of the politics-of-cancer-as-usual have kept you from knowing this, and will continue to do so unless you wake up to this reality." **Lee Cowden MD**

"Almost every patient treated with IL2 (a current conventional cancer treatment) suffered fever, malaise, nausea or vomiting, diarrhoea, sharp drops in blood pressure, skin rashes, breathing difficulties, liver abnormalities and irregularities in blood chemistry. Rosenberg himself details a number of horrifying case histories, and one in particular where the administration of IL2 had precipitated amongst other things, vomiting, swollen joints, lung fluid and 'vascular leak syndrome' where blood would ooze through the vessel walls and collect under the skin." **Steven Rosenberg, The Transformed Cell, Putnam Press, 1992**

"Dr Linus Pauling, often known as the 'Father of Vitamin C' and twice awarded the Nobel Prize, declared that large intakes of up to 10g of the Vitamin Each day aids anti-cancer activity within the body. Pauling was largely derided for making these declarations, but today, large doses of Vitamin C are used by many practitioners for cancer

patients in nutritional therapy, who believe Pauling was right and that the popular nutrient is indispensable to the body in its fight to regain health from cancer." **Phillip Day, Cancer, Why We're Still Dying to Know The Truth, Credence Publications, 2001.**

"Do not let either the medical authorities or the politicians mislead you. Find out what the facts are, and make your own decisions about how to live a happy life and how to work for a better world." **Linus Pauling** http://www.cforyourself.com

The above remarks are representative of a vast library of well-sourced contrary information which sensibly questions the validity and efficacy of conventional cancer treatments based on a huge amount of clinical research and data. Naturally, with all these expensive and patented treatments available to fight cancer, the cancer rates should be going down. They are not. They are increasing.

STAGGERING AMOUNTS
UPHS is locked into the conventional cancer framework - a framework which today, rightly stands accused of achieving no measurable success at all in its approach to the treatment of cancer, immense success in causing widespread, unnecessary death through its application of lethal and highly toxic pharma-radiation treatments, and even greater success in rewarding itself absolutely staggering amounts of money in the whole grisly process. That these cancer corporations have become incredibly wealthy through their 'chemo 'til we drop' approach is a fact which Messrs Siemens, Zeneca, Upjohn, Glaxo, Rhône Poulenc cannot deny.

COMMON SENSE
Pauling was right. We have been seriously misled. Taking the Siemens $multi-million technology as an example. It may well detect certain forms of cancer, but upon detecting it, what then happens? Quite simply, a bewildered, obedient, grateful and unsuspecting cancer sufferer is immediately directed towards the door marked 'iatrogenic (doctor-induced) illness and probable death.' Closer examination of today's orthodox cancer treatments clearly reveals that the conventional path is fraught with toxic danger. But the CEO of UPHS has made it quite clear that *'the Siemens alliance* [one of so many] *is critical to the financial security of UPHS'.*

This is why we will hear no publicly dissenting voices from UPHS as to the horrific realities associated with 20th and 21st century conventional cancer treatments. The corporate big boys' riches must continue to flow.... and a handsome proportion of it into the coffers of the very dependent UPHS, of course, 'to assist in their financial recovery'.

SO WHY THE SLUR ON VITAMIN C?

As has already been stated, conventional cancer treatment represents a $multi-billion a year industry. These vast profits are fiercely protected by the industry giants. But their treatments in no way address the underlying causes of cancer. Cancer is a nutritional/toxic/environmental condition, which, in a great number of instances, can be successfully reversed through the application of a sound nutritional approach and common-sense lifestyle changes. Linus Pauling, dubbed 'the father of Vitamin C', sensibly promoted the benefits of consuming high doses Vitamin C in the prevention of and battle against cancer.

HALF-TRUTHS AND LIES

So why aren't we hearing about these natural treatment successes? Why aren't they being heralded across the world? The answer is money. Despite the multitudinous successes in cancer regression through nutrition, and through extensive application of vital elements such as Vitamin C, Vitamin B17, pancreatic enzymes and other co-factors, Big Pharma is doing all it can to silence these success stories.

To have it become widely known that cancer can be successfully treated without toxic and profitable pharmaceuticals would be catastrophic for its business. Who would continue to purchase these products? What would the Siemens, Glaxo and Upjohn shareholders have to say about that?

To their shame, vested interests are keeping well-proven, non-toxic cancer treatments from the public domain. This is why, under 'cancer treatments', the UPHS website says this of Vitamin B17:

"Several patients displayed symptoms of cyanide poisoning, including muscle weakness and impaired reflexes, or had life-threatening levels of cyanide in their blood. (Laetrile can release cyanide, which is a

highly toxic chemical.) The researchers concluded that Laetrile is not effective as a cancer treatment and is harmful in some cases." [235]

Now read this contrary extract from a radio talk show, featured in Phillip Day's *Cancer, Why We Are Still Dying To Know the Truth*:

Radio host Laurie Lee: *"So this is verified, that Laetrile [B17] can have this positive effect?"*

Dr Ralph Moss: *"We were finding this and yet, we in Public Affairs were told to issue statements to the exact opposite of what we were finding scientifically."*

At the time, Ralph Moss was former Assistant Director of Public Relations at Memorial Sloan Kettering, NY, a leading American conventional cancer research facility.

ONLY A LUNCH AWAY
Of course Laetrile, or Vitamin B17, is not approved by the FDA, but not because it isn't beneficial – it is. No, Vitamin B17 has not been approved by the FDA simply because the FDA has been leaned on. That's the way it goes in the self-preserving, self-serving, conventional cancer business.

To put it bluntly, biddable FDA officials are only a phone call and a golfing lunch away from the NCI and the NIH. A classic example of these conflicts of interests and double standards can be appreciated when one learns that sodium fluoride is also not approved by the FDA due to its toxicity, and yet drug giant Proctor and Gamble and others can market the stuff in their toothpastes, claiming a pharmacological benefit, with complete impunity.

The UPHS statement on Laetrile is a fabrication. Such is the wealth of evidence overturning the conventional stance on Laetrile and Vitamin C, that one can only assume the UPHS statement falls into the following category:

---

[235] http://cancer.med.upenn.edu/pdq_html/6/engl/600093.html

***FALSE SCIENTIFIC RESEARCH 'ENDANGERING THE
PUBLIC'*** - *Independent News, 13ᵗʰ December 2000 - Doctors are
fabricating research results to win grants and advance their careers,
but the medical establishment is failing to protect the public from the
menace of these scientific frauds, a committee of medical editors said
yesterday. Eighty cases of fraudulent research have been detected in
the past four years, and 30 have been investigated in the past year. In
some cases, institutions have covered up wrongdoing to protect
reputations....*

THE NUB OF IT
In an effort to subvert this mass-awakening to the horrors of
conventional cancer treatments, a devious attack on all genuinely
beneficial, natural (and therefore unpatentable) anti-cancer products is
now being waged by a rather worried conventional cancer
establishment. The ever-so-gentle slur on our most vital of vitamins,
Vitamin C, will soon be extended to a wide range of essential minerals
and vitamins.

This is just the beginning of the subtle, but concerted attack. The latest
conventional legislation surrounding the codifying and banning of
efficacious natural treatments is being instituted, purely because there
is no money in these natural treatments for Big Pharma. It is profit
before human health, but couched in respectable-looking, 'sciency'
reports. And this veneer of respectability is fooling the unsuspecting
minions lower down the UPHS research chain.

NAÏVE
The two UPHS officials Credence spoke to regarding Dr Blair's Vitamin
C report were extremely pleasant, open and helpful and displayed no
intention to supply misleading information. But both persons were
entirely locked into their superiors' way of thinking. Media Relations
officer Olivia Fermano was curious as to our interest into who funded
the Vitamin C report. When we pointed out that if Dr Blair's funding
could be traced to a pharmaceutical company producing conventional
cancer treatments, then the results would have to be very seriously
questioned, Ms Fermano was genuinely supportive. *"My goodness!
That is a good question. I will be right back to you."*

Her word-for-word courteous reply, some two minutes later, was as follows: *"You had me genuinely worried for a few minutes there, Sir. But I am pleased to tell you that our funding came directly from the National Institutes for Health.... I am so relieved."*

Ho Hum.

Similarly, Dr Garret Fitzgerald, chair of UPHS Centre for Cancer Pharmacy Department, stated: *"The evidence supporting Vitamin C as a useful adjunct in cancer treatment ranges from scant to non-existent. Linus Pauling's work was framed around a tenuous hypothesis only."*

Whilst the courtesy displayed by Ms Fermano and Dr Fitzgerald is commendable, their naivety is surely the result of them both working in a commercially cocooned workplace, purposefully insulated from the many success stories attributed to non-toxic, metabolic cancer treatments, and from the amazing health benefits accrued from consuming Vitamin C. For an excellent essay on this subject, please visit http://www.vitamincfoundation.org/mega_1_1.html and read an article entitled 'How Much Vitamin C Is Enough?'

For a more in-depth study of the conventional cancer industry, of the very good news concerning non-toxic, proven cancer treatments and of the benefits of Vitamin C, readers are encouraged to visit www.credence.org and take the cancer tour.

Other Book Titles by Credence

Scared Sick of Cancer? Don't Be. Get the Facts... and then get on with your life !

CANCER: WHY WE'RE STILL DYING TO KNOW THE TRUTH
by Phillip Day

For more information on the truth behind cancer and Metabolic Therapy, our world-famous book, *Cancer: Why We're Still Dying to Know the Truth* is the excellent starting point. This overview title exposes the ongoing establishment cover-up over the failure of traditional cancer treatments and explains Metabolic Therapy (Vitamins B17/A&E/enzymes), the controversial treatment for cancer and its prevention. This book further details the amazing track record of nutrition and its role within the simple, combined protocol of Metabolic Therapy. Whether you have cancer, or are exercising prevention for you and your family, PLEASE get educated on this vital issue today.

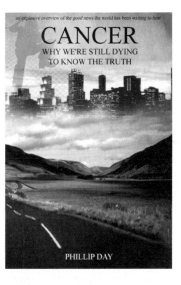

Title: *Cancer: Why We're Still Dying to Know the Truth*
by Phillip Day
ISBN 0-9535012-4-8
First published in April 1999 by Credence Publications
Available at www.credence.org

B17 METABOLIC THERAPY IN THE PREVENTION AND CONTROL OF CANCER
- a technical manual -
compiled by Phillip Day

B17 METABOLIC THERAPY

in the prevention and control of CANCER

a technical manual

compiled by
PHILLIP DAY

From the desks of some of the world's leading cancer scientists comes the empirical proof of Vitamin B17 and its co-factors in the treatment and prevention of cancer. These explosive findings have been the cause of the real cancer war, where vested interests have moved to vilify and denigrate nutrition in order to protect their highly lucrative cancer incomes.

- Find out why 18 'primitive' cultures do not get cancer in their isolated state.
- What three nutritional components have been found vital in the prevention and the treatment of cancer?
- What can you do to change your diet in ways which will give you maximum protection from cancer and other associated ailments?
- Why do animals not get cancer in the wild, yet succumb to it when 'domesticated' by humans?
- Discover the amazing research of Professor John Beard of Edinburgh University and American Biochemist Ernst T Krebs Jr which shows what cancer actually is. Remove your fear of this disease forever.
- Why are huge budgets continually spent on 'fighting the war against cancer' when this information has been in the public domain for 50 years?
- Examine the actual technical theses and trials carried out by doctors and scientists that validate this amazingly simple protocol.

- Find out what you can do today to join the global movement to eradicate cancer from the 21st century!

Phillip Day: *"Now comes the empirical information for doctors, scientists and laymen alike, which can be used at a local, state or global level to eradicate cancer and its heartache from the human race forever. Each of us has a chance today to be great – to remove far from us the greed, entrenched error and ignorance that has allowed cancer to flourish like an evil bloom in our midst. In a sense, cancer will remain around only as long as it takes humankind to achieve that rare level of maturity, when he will treasure his own well-being and that of his friends and loved ones before the tempting lure of wealth, prestige and renown."*

HEALTH WARS

by Phillip Day

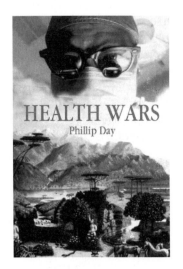

PRESS RELEASE: Western healthcare is now the third leading cause of death in Britain, according to a UK health research organisation. England-based Credence Research, citing statistics which demonstrate that drug-dominated medicine is now the third leading killer in most industrial nations, warns that the true death toll may be far higher than even its reported figures.

Credence Chief Executive Phillip Day states: *"225,000 Americans are killed every year by Western healthcare, according to the American Medical Association. In Britain, the official figure of 40,000 is in reality far higher, if you examine the proper markers. 1 in 5 Australians will be killed every year by their doctors, through incorrect drug-prescribing, botched medical procedures, infections in hospitals and, the main killer, <u>correct</u> drug prescribing. This worldwide allopathic catastrophe is well known to the authorities who, in reality, are unable to do much about it within the current healthcare system, for the reasons we report."*

Credence, whose recently released publication, *Health Wars*, deals with this unsettling phenomenon, states: *"90-95% of the diseases currently killing populations, at least in the industrial nations, are nutritional deficiency and/or toxin related conditions, such as heart disease, cancer, diabetes and stroke. To understand completely why medicine continues to fail with these problems, and worse, be guilty of its own unique slaughter of the citizenry, one need look no further than the fact that doctors receive almost no formal training in nutrition. Thus, doctors are not trained to understand the underlying metabolic problems of at least 90% of diseases, which can be treated effectively, even in their late stages, or completely prevented, using simple, and unfortunately un-patentable nutrition."*

On the toxin disease front, the medical establishment is equally dismissive and trivialises the real chemical and environmental causes, according to Credence. To illustrate why this happens, Day points out that the very industry responsible for producing and selling chemicals, which routinely kill and maim the public, also manufactures the public's medicines. *"Don't expect the chemical industry to gain a morality on this issue overnight. It is hamstrung by stark conflicts of interest. The urgent call for reform needed to prevent further tragedy on the scale we face must come from the public itself."*

On Credence's recently released book, Day declares: *"The purpose of 'Health Wars' is to highlight these problems and to urge citizens to pressure their governments for immediate reform. Compounding its failures, British healthcare has ironically been brought to its knees by the crippling costs of the very drugs and treatments, which have been, and continue to be, the main instigators of these frightening death statistics. Credence has been looking at mortality. But how many citizens out there have been crippled or maimed by healthcare practices, such as vaccinations, errant drug prescribing and unnecessary surgeries? Recent reports show that the NHS must budget every year for at least £2.8 billion in compensation claims alone. That's enough to build and fully staff 28 new hospitals every twelve months."*

Credence states that medical science has known for years that the answers to heart disease, cancer, stroke and other illnesses lie completely in nutrition and lifestyle changes, not radical surgeries, toxic drugs or radiation. To prove this point, the company cites at least 18 cultures alive today who do not apparently suffer from these health problems. *"Interestingly,"* Day elaborates, *"we tend to call these peoples 'primitive' and 'less developed'. But they know enough about nutrition to ensure that they survive in sterling health, in many cases to over 100 years of age. The authorities know this too, and do nothing. Why? Because Western healthcare today is a multi-trillion-dollar industry worldwide, and you cannot pay CEO salaries and shareholder dividends using apples, oranges and chemical-free, organic vegetation."*

Day believes that health reform is inevitable, and that the public can do much to precipitate the process by getting educated and politically active: *"A proper healthcare industry must have nutritional education at its heart,"* he states. *"This is the most basic body science. We are what we eat. But the people will have to fight a war with their industrial and political peers first, in order to secure the return of their unalienable right to drink fresh, uncontaminated water, to eat fresh, uncontaminated food and to breathe fresh, uncontaminated air."*

Title: *Health Wars*
by Phillip Day
ISBN 1-904015-01-8 (325 pages)
First edition published June 2001 by Credence Publications
Available at www.credence.org

FOOD FOR THOUGHT

compiled by Phillip Day

Need a guide on where to go with your food? What better way to embrace the dietary concepts laid down in *Cancer:Why We're Still Dying to Know the Truth* and *Health Wars* than to obtain a copy of our official recipe book.

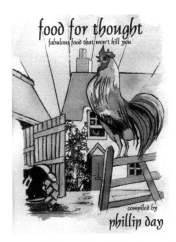

This delightful guide takes you through the main concepts of acid/alkali, Vitamin B17 dishes, the proper combining of foods, the problems with meat and dairy in excessive amounts, fruit consumption techniques, a host of detox menus, 5-10% meat and dairy recipes, snacks, pro-active sickness dieting, children's dishes and proper supplementation. Whether you are suffering or just want to make a change for your extended future, sensible nutrition comes to life in *Food For Thought*, bringing you the most delicious foods that WON'T KILL YOU!

Title: *Food for Thought*
Compiled by Phillip Day
ISBN 1-904015-04-2
First published in August 2001 by Credence Publications
Available at www.credence.org

PLAGUE, PESTILENCE AND THE PURSUIT OF POWER

by Steven Ransom

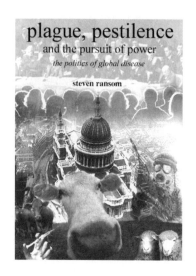

Almost every day, it seems, we are hearing reports of some 'highly infectious' disease breaking out somewhere across the world - the recent flu pandemics, AIDS decimating Africa, tuberculosis on the rise again, measles, and meningitis on the increase. And in the animal kingdom, we've seen Bovine Spongiform Encephalopathy (BSE), poultry flu, swine fever, more BSE and now foot and mouth, wreaking havoc across our countryside. One could be forgiven for thinking that we are quite literally surrounded by virulent illness. But not everything is as it seems – not by a long way.

In this book, we discover that these so-called 'epidemics' are NOT the deadly illnesses we have been led to believe by our respective governments, national papers and news programs. With all the above-mentioned illnesses, the facts being disseminated have been grossly misleading, accompanied, in many instances, by a deliberate intent to scare and deceive. Welcome to the shocking world of the politically manufactured epidemic - the 'psycho-plague'.

The formula is quite simple. Using the mainstream media as their chosen vehicle for change, powerful vested interests are deliberately instigating national and international fearsome headlines. Through these channels, the problem – the epidemic – the psycho-plague, is manufactured. A crisis has now been firmly embedded into the mind of the populace. **"We must have a solution!"** we cry. Lo and behold, a governmental/corporate solution is speedily proffered.

In reality, the epidemic needing 'swift state intervention' has been nothing more than a Trojan Horse either for creating immense profit for various pharmaceutical industries or, as we shall discover, for ushering in unsavoury, global super-state ideology. Throughout this whole process, we are being taught what to think about health and disease, but not how.

In examining the facts laid out before us, we soon realise that our battle is not so much against pathological disease, as against corrupt and self-serving desires, birthed in the minds of man. This book contains the supporting evidence to make this case. You are invited to consider the evidence for yourself.

But this book also maps out a positive way forward. For, in discovering the true nature and causes of these 'epidemics', a longer lasting remedy can now be planned for the future.

Plague, Pestilence and the Pursuit of Power is dedicated to those who want to find out what really goes on behind the closed doors of Big Business and Big Government and to those who wish to see truth reign in conventional science and medicine.

Title: *Plague, Pestilence and the Pursuit of Power*
by Steven Ransom
ISBN 0-9535012-8-0 (205 pages)
First published in June 2001 by Credence Publications
Available at www.credence.org

All titles can also be obtained from the distributor whose details are in the *Contacts!* section of this book.

WORLD WITHOUT AIDS

by Steven Ransom & Phillip Day

WORLD
WITHOUT
AIDS

Steven Ransom
&
Phillip Day

One of the greatest scandals in medicine today surrounds the classification of AIDS as an infectious disease. The supposed pathogen, human immunodeficiency virus (HIV), despite much fanfare and fear-mongering, has never been isolated according to any recognised and appropriate scientific procedure. And so, from a scientific standpoint, HIV can be deemed not to exist. Since Dr Robert Gallo's so-called 'discovery of HIV' in 1984 (at which he displayed a fake 'image' for which he was later convicted of science fraud), no empirical proof for the existence of HIV has ever been furnished to the scientific establishment. Monetary rewards for 'The Missing Virus' remain uncollected by the conventional scientific community for a properly isolated HI virus, according to all the normal rules.

All the evidence shows that immune suppression ('AIDS') in the Western World is primarily brought on by long-term recreational or pharmaceutical drug toxicity **AND IS NOT INFECTIOUS OR SEXUALLY TRANSMITTED**. So-called Third World or 'African' 'AIDS' is nothing more than the cynical reclassification of diseases that have always killed Africans, namely: dysentery, cholera, malnutrition, TB, malaria, typhoid and parasitic infections, brought on by the frequently contaminated water supplies which Africans and inhabitants of other nations are forced to tolerate. To add to this injustice, Africans are almost always classified as 'AIDS carriers' by the authorities through visual diagnosis only. This arbitrary, World Health Organisation-approved method of diagnosis is known as the Bangui method.

In order to be deemed an AIDS carrier under Bangui, one need only be suffering from diarrhoea, fever and demonstrate a 10% weight loss over a two-month period. These symptoms can of course relate to

208

almost all of the above-mentioned diseases that were (and still are) common across Africa prior to all the dramatic AIDS headlines. Illnesses that are relatively simple to treat have now been cynically clustered under the AIDS umbrella. The collective impact of this manoeuvre serves only to reinforce the errant belief that HIV is decimating Africa and other poorer nations. It also gives more credibility to the growing number of reports that AIDS is re-emerging in the West.

In the West, AIDS is hardly less scandalous. Many unwitting victims are drawn into the AIDS nightmare by inadvertently triggering a 'positive' on one of two main tests given to patients today. The ELISA (Enzyme-Linked Immuno-Absorbent Assay) and Western Blot tests are designed to highlight the presence of the supposed HIV, not by identifying the virus itself, but by indicating the presence of antibodies in the blood allegedly unique to, and stimulated by the virus. But as we have already discovered, all the diagnostic methods employed by the recognised laboratories are far from specific. Prominent AIDS researcher Christine Maggiore, herself a victim of these fraudulent tests, states the major problem as follows:

"Both tests are non-specific to HIV antibodies and are highly inaccurate. Non-specific means that these tests respond to a great number of non-HIV antibodies, microbes, bacteria and other conditions that are often found in the blood of normal, healthy people. A reaction to any one of these other antibodies and conditions will result in an HIV positive diagnosis. A simple illness like a cold or the flu can cause a positive reading on an HIV test. A flu shot or other vaccine can also create positive results. Having or having had herpes or hepatitis may produce a positive test, as can a vaccination for hepatitis B. Exposure to diseases such as tuberculosis and malaria commonly cause false positive results, as do the presence of tape worms and other parasites. Conditions such as alcoholism, liver disease and blood that is highly oxidated through drug use may be interpreted as the presence of HIV antibodies. Pregnancy and prior pregnancy can also cause a positive result." [236]

---

[236] Maggiore, Christine, *What if Everything You Thought You Knew About AIDS Was Wrong?* Alive and Well, Studio City, CA 90604, USA

The triggering of an HIV positive will lead invariably to prescriptions for the deadly cell toxins AZT, ddI and other 'HIV' drugs, which have an appalling history of causing the very immune deficiencies they were supposedly designed to prevent. South African barrister Anthony Brink remarks:

"In truth, AZT makes you feel like you're dying. That's because on AZT you are. How can a deadly cell toxin conceivably make you feel better as it finishes you, by stopping your cells from dividing, by ending this vital process that distinguishes living things from dead things? Not for nothing does AZT come with a skull and cross-bones label when packaged for laboratory use." [237]

And indeed that is the case. With a skull and cross-bones on the outer label and a reminder to wear suitable protective clothing when handling, the inner contents of the AZT packaging include the following side-effects advisory notice:

WHOLE BODY: abdominal pain, back pain, body odour, chest pain, chills, edema of the lip, fever, flu symptoms, hyperalgesia.
CARDIOVASCULAR: syncope, vasodilation.
GASTROINTESTINAL: bleeding gums, constipation, diarrhoea, dysphagia, edema of the tongue, eructation, flatulence, mouth ulcer, rectal haemorrhage.
HAEMIC AND LYMPHATIC: lymphadenopathy.
MUSCULOSKELETAL: arthralgia, muscle spasm, tremor, twitch.
NERVOUS: anxiety, confusion, depression, dizziness, emotional lability, loss of mental acuity, nervousness, paresthesia, somnolence, vertigo.
RESPIRATORY: cough, dyspnea, epistaxis, hoarseness, pharyngitis, rhinitis, sinusitis.
SKIN: rash, sweat, urticaria.
SPECIAL SENSES: amblyopia, hearing loss, photophobia, taste perversion.
UROGENITAL: dysuria, polyuria, urinary frequency, urinary hesitancy.

---

[237] Brink, Anthony, *AZT and Heavenly Remedies*, Rethinking AIDS Homepage: www.rethinkingaids.com

Phillip Day spent eight years in Los Angeles and San Francisco working with those deemed HIV positive by the medical establishment. In all cases, he reports, their plight could be laid at the door of excessive lifestyles, recreational or pharmaceutical drug terrorism and a general lack of education surrounding the true nature and causes of immune deficiency. Their sure and ready remedy was to move towards wellness with a properly constructed regimen of sound nutrition and supplementation. The full Credence report is contained in *World Without AIDS*, the result of 15 years' research into this tragically misunderstood realm of medical fraud, injustice and error.

It seems though that with these profitable AIDS treatments, the fraud, injustice and error is set to continue. A mandatory AIDS vaccine is looming.

REPORT PREDICTS MASSIVE RESISTANCE TO MANDATORY AIDS VACCINE - *Wes Vernon, NewsMax, 24th June, 2001 - A new report predicts massive resistance to a mandatory AIDS vaccine that is coming to the US in the next few years. Millions of parents would refuse to have their children vaccinated by any variation of an HIV/AIDS shot, the Committee to Protect Medical Freedom said at a news conference Wednesday. Jim Turner, a Washington attorney and expert on the swine flu vaccine scandal of the 1970s, lent his support, as did Barbara Lee Fisher, co-founder and president of the National Vaccine Information Center. The thrust of the report, written by Clifford Kincaid, is that there's big money in rushing an AIDS vaccine to market, some of it tied up in conflict-of-interest questions involving the promoters and their connections with companies that stand to benefit.*

Barbara Loe Fisher, co-founder of the National Vaccine Information Center, reports that a member of the federal committee that recommends vaccines for children had said that an AIDS vaccine would be tested and then forced on all 12-year-old children. Neal Halsey, M.D., chairman of the American Academy of Pediatrics (AAP) Committee on Infectious Diseases, reminded HIV vaccine researchers and developers at a meeting in February 1997 of an advisory committee of the federal Centers for Disease Control that CDC plans to target 11- to 12-year-old children for "universal application" of an HIV vaccine.

The Kincaid study says, "...babies are being used as guinea pigs now." The National Institute for Allergy and Infectious Diseases, under the auspices of the federal Department of Health and Human Services, is sponsoring an HIV vaccine test on babies born to HIV-infected women." [238]

If this wasn't bad enough, every expectant mothers in the UK is now being recommended to take an 'HIV' test. In some states in the US, the test is mandatory. Submitting to this test will result in these women standing a chance of being deemed HIV positive, simply because of the mother's heightened levels of antibody activity picked up by these tests. The resultant medication is as catastrophic to the baby as it is to the mother. For this reason, Credence has issued the following advisory leaflet for the urgent attention of all expectant mothers and all those planning to start a family. The leaflet is available in printer-friendly format at www.credence.org

* * * * *

HEALTH WARNING TO EXPECTANT MOTHERS

If you have recently become pregnant, you will be recommended to take an HIV test as part of a standardised ante-natal care package.[239] This test is highly inaccurate and remains scientifically unproven. It should be refused on the following grounds.

1) All manufacturers of these tests include the following or similar disclaimer with their test kits: "At present, there is no recognised standard for establishing the presence or absence of antibodies to HIV-1 and HIV- 2 in human blood."[240]

---

[238] The full report can be found at:
http://www.newsmax.com/archives/articles/2001/6/20/152903.shtml
[239] Refer to "Review of antenatal testing services", NHS Regional Office, London, UK Dept of Health. Recommending the HIV test became UK national policy in July 1999, and is now mandatory in some US states.
[240] The above disclaimer is included in all Abbott 'AXSYM' Aids tests at the time of writing, the world's leading supplier of AIDS test kits.

2) The reason for this disclaimer is because the AIDS test does not measure the presence of a virus.[241] The AIDS test has been designed to detect levels of antibody activity in the blood. Antibody activity in the blood stream is a normal occurrence in humans, but is being misinterpreted by the AIDS test as indicative of the presence of HIV.

3) As a result of this misinterpretation, healthy individuals are being wrongly diagnosed as HIV positive. Since this information has come to light, in excess of 60 different medical conditions have been recorded that can give rise to a false HIV positive reading. These separate conditions include flu, flu vaccination, malaria, tetanus vaccination, Hepatitis A and B, Hepatitis vaccinations, alcohol and drug use, recent viral infections and even pregnancy.[242] Receiving a spurious but emotionally devastating diagnosis of HIV positive will prompt your doctor to recommend a course of anti-HIV drugs. Known as protease inhibitors or anti-retrovirals, these drugs are highly toxic. They have the well-documented capacity to harm the mother, and also severely to deform and even kill the unborn child. [243]

The current level of spending on AIDS drugs in the Western World is phenomenal. So too are the profits enjoyed by the AIDS drug manufacturers. As a result, the information contained in this advisory leaflet is largely being ignored by the medical establishment. Sadly, this is not an unexpected reaction. The pursuit of profit at the expense of health, the wilful employment of flawed medical procedures, the administration of dangerously toxic drugs to expectant mothers, the disregard for the plight of thousands upon thousands of wrongly diagnosed people, and a refusal by the medical establishment to listen

---

[241] Monetary rewards offered to leading organisations within the scientific community by concerned organisations for reasonable evidence that HIV exists remain uncollected.

[242] Johnson, Christine, *Continuum Magazine*, September 1996. Maggiore, Christine, *What if Everything You Knew about AIDS was Wrong?* An Alive and Well Publication, April 2000. Ransom & Day, *World Without AIDS*, Credence Publications, July 2000.

[243] Kumar et al, *Journal of Acquired Immune Deficiency Syndromes*, 7; 1034-9, 1994. *JAMA Journal of American Medical Association*, Jan 5th 2000, Incidence of liver damage. *World Without AIDS*. AZT and enlarged craniums in infants. Refer to www.virusmyth.com for a more comprehensive list of scientific references which catalogue the damage caused by AIDS drugs.

to sound contrary evidence or to admit medical negligence - all these are the hallmarks of that once-respected drug, thalidomide. Do not allow either yourself or your child to face the possibility of becoming another heartbreaking medical statistic.

WORLD WITHOUT AIDS

World Without AIDS dismantles one of the world's greatest fears and lays bare the deceit, fraudulent science and needless fearmongering that lie at the heart of this supposed global epidemic. Over ten years in the making, this impeccably researched book gives an eye-opening account of what vested interests can get away with, given a trusting public, an almost limitless supply of money and scant scruples. It also explains the non-existence of HIV, the bankruptcy of the HIV test, the real causes of immune suppression, the AIDS-devastating-Africa myth and the appalling dangers of the establishment-approved medications prescribed to those who have been written off as 'HIV positive'.

Title: *World Without AIDS*
by Steve Ransom and Phillip Day
ISBN 0-9535012-5-6
First published in June 2000 by Credence Publications
Available through credence.org

Campaign for Truth in Medicine

"a force for change"

WHAT IS CTM?

Campaign for Truth in Medicine is a worldwide organisation dedicated to pressing for change in areas of science and medicine where entrenched scientific error, ignorance or vested interests are costing lives. Its ranks comprise doctors, scientists, researchers, biochemists, politicians, industry executives and countless members of the world public, all of whom have made one

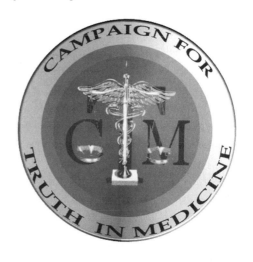

observation in common. They have recognised that, in certain key areas of global disease, drug treatments and overall healthcare philosophy, the medical, chemical and political establishments are pursuing the wrong course with the maximum of precision, even when their own legitimate and erudite scientific research has illustrated the dangers of pursuing these courses.

CTM BACKS ITS PEOPLE'S CHARTER

CTM's People's Charter catalogues these key problem areas - for example AIDS, cancer, heart disease and vaccinations - where the preponderance of evidence demonstrates severe cause for concern over deadly errors in basic science, resulting in needless loss of life. CTM's charter also highlights industry's every-day use of potentially harmful contaminants and biohazards, such as toothpaste's sodium fluoride, shampoo's sodium lauryl sulphate and cosmetic's propylene glycol, which have long been linked to long-term serious health risks and death. CTM's purpose is to present this damning evidence to its members, to the public at large and to the establishments and individuals involved in these errors, in order to press for immediate change and cessation of their use for the benefit of humanity. The

People's Charter is periodically amended to reflect current issues and new areas of concern.

CTM STANDS FOR TRUTH

For decades members of the public and a significant proportion of their medical and scientific professionals have become increasingly angry and frustrated at what they see as establishment indifference and even downright hostility towards much-needed changes in healthcare, especially in areas where the proven solution is substantially less profitable than the current status quo.

PROMOTING THE TRUTH

CTM believes in promoting the truth in these matters, thereby exposing those morally bankrupt and compromised politicians, corporations and individuals responsible. This method of action is viewed as a top priority. CTM is dedicated to pushing for immediate change, in order that immediate relief from many of the diseases and their causes, currently afflicting us, may be implemented, the remedies for which, in certain cases, have been a matter of existing scientific knowledge for decades.

The Journal of the American Medical Association (JAMA) implicitly reports that western healthcare, along with its drugs, treatments and hospitals, is now the third leading cause of death in the United States, next to heart disease and cancer. If we examine this astonishing fact, also highlighted by US consumer advocate Ralph Nader in the early 1990's, we come to realise that the Western healthcare paradigm is adopted by almost all developed nations and many other developing countries around the world. Thus this tragic statistic of iatrogenic death can be fairly considered to be global in application.

This would be serious enough on its own, yet the true extent of this orthodox medical catastrophe is unfortunately far more devastating. Western medical establishments are in possession of key life-saving information that can immediately and drastically reduce current and future global incidences of cancer, heart disease, AIDS and other treatable, non-fatal conditions. But in almost all cases these institutions have chosen neither to adopt these measures, train their healthcare practitioners in these practices, nor publicize the latter to a generally trusting world populace. Thus these government personnel and their associated medical luminaries, who have wilfully kept this life-saving information from their doctors and the public, may justifiably be exposed for becoming the leading cause of death across the planet today.

CTM STANDS FOR DIRECT ACTION
CTM believes that, in certain cases, legitimate direct action is warranted against these institutions and individuals to halt their wilful and harmful actions and hold them to account. In these circumstances, CTM calls upon its membership to organise and act in a unified, lawful and mature fashion to bring these matters to the attention of the mass communications media, government leaders and heads of state through demonstrations and other appropriate action. CTM is dedicated to being part of the people's movement in this regard; a powerful and irresistible force for change, compelling vital reform TODAY for a safer and healthier world for our children and children's children.

CTM IS FREE FROM VESTED INTEREST FUNDING
Through its network of worldwide professional contacts, CTM has constant access to well-researched information on key health issues. CTM brings its members highly readable and jargon-free information, such as that contained in this book.

CTM HAS ALL THE NECESSARY CONTACTS
...at local and central government/corporate level, responsible for particular health legislation and legislative change. Names, addresses, contact details and relevant template letters are supplied with all CTM newsletters.

CTM IS A HEALTH ADVOCACY ORGANISATION
with purpose and direction. It is a conduit through which the individual minority voice can become a powerful and respected, collective majority voice for change.

WHAT YOU CAN DO NOW

CTM invites you to visit its web-site to learn more about how you can join this worldwide movement FOR FREE and receive regular bulletins and further information on these fascinating subjects as they develop. Be part of a different future. One that celebrates life!

**Campaign for Truth in Medicine
PO Box 3
Tonbridge,
Kent,
TN 12 9ZY UK
e-mail: info@campaignfortruth.com
www.campaignfortruth.com**

Contacts! Contacts! Contacts!

If you wish to purchase more copies of this book or find out where you may obtain any of the products or materials discussed in this book, please use the contact details below:

US Auto Orders: (309) 416 8714
UK Orders: (01622) 832386
Int'l Orders: +44 1622 832386
UK Fax: (01622) 833314
www.credence.org
e-mail: sales@credence.org

HEALTH REVIEW AND FREE INFORMATION PACK

What other book entitles you to a free magazine subscription and regular e-mail updates completely free? If you have not received these and have purchased this book, contact us on the above numbers.

Credence also sends hundreds of free information packs throughout the world every month to those who have requested them either for themselves or for interested friends and relatives. Those who receive such packs will receive our seasonal magazine *Health Review*, informing the reader of the latest developments on this and other interesting health topics. If you would like to take advantage of this service, please supply the relevant mailing address details to our head office address below:

Credence Publications
PO Box 3
TONBRIDGE
Kent TN12 9ZY
England
infopack@credence.org

ECLUB BULLETINS

Twice each month, the Campaign for Truth in Medicine sends out the EClub Internet bulletin to thousands of subscribers worldwide. This highly informative e-mail newsletter is available FREE to customers who have purchased this book or who have requested EClub. This online bulletin contains the latest news and research on cancer and other vital health topics. DO NOT BE WITHOUT THIS GREAT RESOURCE! If you wish to subscribe, log on to the Campaign site at www.campaignfortruth.com and click the 'Join CTM' tab to complete your free application.

Index

About The Author

Bill Kellner-Read qualified as a dentist from King's College Hospital, London in 1977. After a brief time as a junior dental officer, he moved into general practice. The routine of drilling and filling soon sent Bill looking for more interesting and absorbing areas of dentistry: *"After a while, fillings are about as interesting as watching paint dry, except that paint comes in more colours!"*

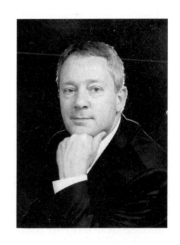

In his practice, he saw more and more people who suffered headaches. Some were self-inflicted after a game of rugby. Others were genuine, daily headaches. These were people who were given Valium and told to live with their pain - people who, for many days at a time, were shut in a darkened room in misery, waiting for the latest episode to pass. This area was to become the focus of a long career, treating chronic pain of dental origin. The Pankey Institute in Miami, Dr Harold Gelb DDS of New York, Dr Richard Pertes DDS of the School of Medicine and Dentistry, New Jersey and Dr Aelred Fonder DDS of Rock Falls, Illinois – all these people and organisations and more, were instrumental in Bill's early education in this field.

The whole area of head and neck pain dovetails into the overall concept of biological dentistry. Bill began to look at the materials he was using in practice that could adversely affect his patients. Fluoride compounds, mercury and root fillings came under scrutiny, as did oral hygiene products and the area of nutrition.

It was not long before Bill was introduced to the health concepts of Hans Selye, an Austrian-Hungarian endocrinologist whose famous and revolutionary concept of stress opened countless new avenues of treatment for disease. Selye was Founder and Director of the Institute of Experimental Medicine and Surgery at the University of Montreal and has been regarded as 'the father of stress'.[244] His concepts have been a great help in understanding the complexity and accumulation of stressors that ultimately bring about the downfall of the body.

Bill's professional life has taken him from England to Australia and back. He has sought, learned and lectured on the myriad answers to questions that have been posed by patients earnestly seeking better health.

Completion of this book finds the author back in England in private practice, still leading the cause for better health through dentistry. Bill believes that the dentist of the future will recognise that he/she works within a speciality of medicine; that the mouth is a part of the whole and that the many conditions, currently being treated by the medical profession without any dental intervention, will one day include dentistry in their diagnosis.

Dr Bill Read: *"Medicine and dentistry are missing out on the full potential of looking at the structural, chemical and emotional stressors that come from the mouth and supporting structures. These stressors are currently blighting the lives of many. This book is written to address some of these issues and open the way for further understanding, self-help and the pursuance of good health.*

Through nutrition, dental corrections, eradication of harmful dental products and plenty of pure water, health issues that have ruined lives can be reversed.

In short, the seemingly insignificant area of the mouth can play a truly significant role in the overall span of health and wellbeing."

---

[244] Selye, Hans, *The Stress of My Life*, ibid.

— Notes —

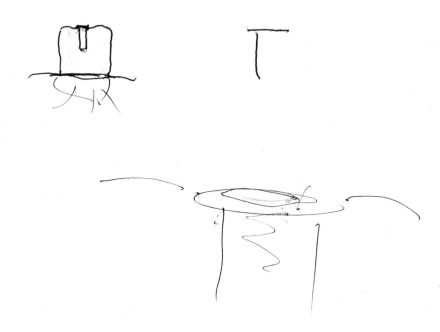